How to get the most from your doctor's visit

To order additional copies, please contact us.
BookSurge, LLC
www.booksurge.com
1-866-308-6235
orders@booksurge.com

MAHMOUD
ELGHOROURY, MD, FAAP

HOW TO GET
THE MOST FROM
YOUR DOCTOR'S
VISIT

2006

How to get the most from your doctor's visit

CHAPTER ONE
Introduction

The Center for Disease Control estimates people make 535 million visits per year to primary care physicians. Of these visits, almost half are due to acute illness (41.5%), with the second most common reason being chronic illness (29.6%) and the third preventive care (23.3%.) Logical prediction will tell you the number of these visits will keep on climbing year after year, probably at an accelerated pace as more of the baby boomers retire and have more time to take care of their health.

But this raises a question: *Did each patient get the most benefit out of each visit?*

I've asked people, and the answer I got from many was *not really*. I listened to friends who complained they hated going to the doctor, with each having a different reason. "Such a waste of time," one said, *I spent a whole day just to get an antibiotic prescription*. Another was frustrated because his doctor does not listen to him long enough. A lot of people reported, "I went to three doctors and each one gave me a different opinion." Another good one is "*My doctor does not know what is wrong with me*."

When I listen to people in coffee shops or malls complaining of bad experiences at their doctor's office, I wonder: is it a lack of resources? But this can't be, as billions upon billions of dollars are spent on health care every year. Not enough people committed to the job? There are millions who work hard every day in many health organizations to help others get better. Yet we're still not satisfied.

In my opinion, major improvement is necessary in the face-to-face encounter between the patient (health care consumer) and the physician (health care provider.) Each one of us should work harder to get better results from that encounter. As basic and elementary as it sounds, each one of those encounters is either a waste or a benefit. The face-to-face encounter between the consumer and the provider of the service is the core of health care.

Yet whose responsibility is it to educate health care consumers? Television commercials are doing a great job introducing new, expensive medications whether you need them or not. They also MOTIVATE you to go to your doctor, not to benefit from her expertise, but to tell her what medicine is good for you. In 30 seconds you learned that you have an allergy that can be best treated with that new wonder drug, so just go to your doctor and ask for his signature on a pre-written prescription—or better yet, call him on the phone. After all, *why would you want to waste time going there?*

I believe it's the responsibility of the people who know to educate the people who do not. We need to pass our knowledge and experience to others so they can benefit from the good and learn from the bad. The future generation must build on past practices to achieve better ones. That was the attitude I learned while in pediatric residency training. We owe it to everyone who is willing to listen to what we—the fieldworkers—have to say. By educating the consumers, the quality will go up while the cost will go down.

A car would cost $100,000 and break every month if it was not for the informed buyers who looked around, compared, and made a choice, as well as the engineers who cared to make better cars and the field workers who kept on raising the standards year after year. Perhaps informed health care consumers will be the ones to force a change rather than the politicians and accountants.

But what is an informed health care consumer? A consumer is one who will not accept a 3-minute encounter with her primary care physician after waiting two hours in the waiting room. A consumer who expects thoughtful, not a knee-jerk reflex kind of care. A consumer who will admire her doctor not for the car he drives, but for the care he delivers.

I once heard a confession of a general pediatrician. He was presenting a large-scale community project to which he'd devoted himself after retiring very early from health care. As he told us about his background, he said, "I used to work in an upper class Chicago suburb with a 4-pediatrician group making a lot of money. But after years of this high paying job, I couldn't take it any more. Because I was forced to see a patient every 3 minutes, from 8 AM to 5 PM I would see 90 patients."

He resigned and committed himself to volunteer community work. As that was in the mid 1990s, you would hope things are different now, but maybe or maybe not. If not, even if you as the health care consumer don't force a change, others will do it for you. Either way the change is inevitable. Why not be one of the first to benefit by becoming an informed consumer now?

My goal in writing this book is to enable you to get the most benefit from a visit to your primary care physician. In other words, I would like to help you be a better consumer of health care.

Is that goal important? Think of the time and money that can be saved for you and your family. These savings will extend to health insurance companies that keep raising their monthly premiums to cope with expenses.

In particular, prudent financing of health care for the aging population needs every consumer to participate actively in the process. I regularly get cost reports from multiple health insurance companies, and I know we can do a better job both as providers and consumers. It is not enough to educate physicians, as for the best outcome in an encounter between a provider (physician) and a consumer (patient), both parties should be educated.

But what about the abundant book supply on health conditions, including obesity, diabetes, and mental disorders? Don't they inform you? These are great educational supplements if you have already seen your doctor and listened to her advice as they can be part of the care plans you receive from your doctor.

But alone they're not substitutes for a physician's observations and guidance.

Definitions and clarifications

Before you begin reading, I would like to clarify some terms. When I use the word *you* in this book, it really means each one of us. Because I go to my primary care physician as much as anybody else, I use it sometimes to replace the word *patient,* which is a 14th- century word that means an individual waiting, or under medical care and treatment. *You* may also replace the terms *health care customer* or *consumer.*

A primary care physician is your personal doctor, your gatekeeper to the wonderland of health care. She is the one you go to for your annual check up and immunizations as well as when you have a sore throat. Years ago when the HMO fantasy of improving health and reducing cost was at a peak, most physicians wanted to be listed as primary care providers. Now that the trend is reversing and HMO enrollment is receding, almost every primary care physician wants to specialize.

In any case, a specialist is a doctor who focuses his practice on a specific body organ, e.g. cardiologists on the heart, nephrologists on the kidney, dermatologists on the skin, and so on. In contrast, a primary care physician is interested in the big picture—ALL of you from head to toe, inside and out.

The health insurance industry offers three basic options to consumers: Traditional or FFS (fee for service) plans, HMO (health maintenance organization) plans, and PPO (preferred provider organization) plans.

The traditional option allows you to pick and choose any doctor to go to, so whether you choose to go to a primary care physician or a specialist such as a cardiologist, the insurance company will pay. They also don't force you to go to your primary care physician first in order to see a specialist.

On the opposite side, an HMO plan is a restricted one featuring structured networks. You have to select a primary care physician (sometime called the gatekeeper), and you can only visit (be referred to) a specialist in the plan's network of health care providers. After you sign the contract, you will be given a directory book and manual. You are bound to follow their rules or pay the entire charge out of your own pocket.

The PPO is a crossover between the other two models. This plan provides you with a directory of physicians for whom the plan will pay more of the cost should you opt to see one, but you also can select an outside/out-of-network health provider at the risk of paying more yourself. This option is appealing to many who want to save money, yet have more choices.

The last statistics I reviewed grouped Americans with health insurance into five categories: 51% obtained health insurance from their employers, 15% through the federal government (Medicare), 15% through their state government (Medicaid), and approximately 4% buy their own health insurance. Of course we should never forget the almost 45 million who have no health insurance, even though 8 out of 10 have jobs or live in a household with someone who has one.

The other piece of relevant information here that may impact how much you pay for a doctor's visit is the amount of dollars your insurance will classify as deductible or out-of-pocket. The general rule is the lower your monthly insurance premium, the higher your deductibles and co-payments will be, and vice versa.

PCP Visit is the Best Deal

I was not surprised when my friend told me, "The vice-president of the hospital said during the meeting that pediatricians are *at the bottom of the food chain*." The hospital employed many physicians in different specialties, but because pediatricians (as primary care providers) didn't generate much income to the hospital (their employer), they didn't have much clout to speak of, unlike heart specialists or plastic surgeons who generate millions of dollars in revenue. For every year I was employed at that hospital, there was always resentment among us pediatricians. We worked so hard, yet the losses kept on mounting.

In an article published in the March 2006 *Infectious Diseases in Children* journal addressing poor payment issues as to general pediatricians, Richard Lander, MD, who works with the American Academy of Pediatrics section on administration and practice management, highlighted a common problem. Managed care organizations or HMOs actually deny payments of certain services to primary care physicians (such as pediatricians) if they determine these services should be provided by specialists!

He suggested to the general pediatricians that they argue their case with the managed care organization medical director: *"You could advise him/her of the consequences. You could send those patients to the pediatric pulmonologist (lung specialist) or to the emergency department. We are much more cost-effective than emergency department doctors"* He continued, *"Pediatricians should not forget that usually we are a less expensive alternative for providing care."*

Do you need proof that we (primary care providers) are the least expensive and most affordable deal in health care? Ask any hospital administrator how much profit or (loss) they generate from primary care clinics (excluding emergency rooms), as most of them would love to cut off the primary care clinics they sponsor because almost all of them are losing money right and left. Most of the hospital's profit comes from expensive procedures, whether in radiology such as MRI or in surgery such as hip replacements, as that's where the money is. Hospital administrator keep primary care physicians and clinics open at a loss so they can feed in patients (customers) to their staff specialists who perform these profitable procedures in the hospital.

For example, my daughter visited a cardiologist for a condition I manage every day in my practice, but my wife insisted on a specialist opinion. I charge between $65 to $110 (depending on if an EKG is needed.) The cardiologist visit's final cost was $1000 with the outcome being exactly the same. I listened to every word he said to my daughter, which matched every word I had told her before. But my wife was pleased that the same recommendation came from a specialist.

The director of the Johns Hopkins University Primary Care Policy Center, Barbara Starfield, MD, MPH, wrote in her article "The Importance of Primary Care to Health" in the medical reporter:

"It is not only having health insurance that influences the likelihood of good health. The quality of services that are available to people also counts. Most people in the U.S. think that having free access to high-powered specialists assures them best quality of care. Unfortunately, this is not the case."

Supply and demand

You may think it is the supply and demand formula that drives compensation, with more primary care physicians meaning greater competition and less compensation, while fewer specialty physicians means they make more money, but you would be dead wrong. In 2004, the number of specialists in the United States exceeded the number of primary care physicians by 176,509. In other words, there were 1.8 specialists for every primary care physician. This can only happen in America, I tell you—enjoy it while it lasts. Take advantage of your primary care physician before the system changes.

The future health care changes may not accommodate the discrepancy between primary care physician and specialists. This is not just my own personal opinion: look at any recommendation from health care groups regional or national, political or financial, as they have all learned from their research data that optimum utilization of primary care is essential for any progress in the health care system.

That's why I'm confident the best deal in health care today is a visit to your primary care physician, which I will prove to you as well by the end of the book. Just bear with me here. But before I get started, let me introduce to you some of your Primary Care Physician credentials.

Credentials and the spinal tap.

Your primary care physician (provider) must successfully finish hundreds of college credit hours to obtain a doctoral degree in human medicine. She spent many years after high school in a competitive grueling scientific educational environment to obtain that medical degree. She also had to undergo a merciless residency program where she was not only trained under strict supervision to diagnose, care for and prevent illnesses, but was also subject to abuse by her superiors who enjoyed her inferior rank, peers who wanted to dump more work on her, and nurses who got their revenge in advance knowing that this resident one day will graduate and be able to boss them around. That is not all: if you cared to hear the stories about how patients give the medical residents a hard time, it would fill your ears for years.

One of my colleagues during his residency had to carry his medical license in his wallet at all times to show it to one of the patients who needed frequent blood draws and would only trust licensed physicians to perform them. I had a mother insisting that my attending chief neurologist perform the spinal tap procedure on her child rather than me (a pediatric resident at the time.) The child had been admitted to the hospital at night, and the spinal tap procedure was requested by the neurologist as part of the child's investigation. My attending went to the mother the following morning and told her, "This pediatric resident performs a lot more spinal tap procedures per day than me, so your child is better off if my resident does it."

So you are getting a smart doctor (supposedly) with long years of serious education and training. How much are you paying for her services?

The vast majority of us will pay our primary care physician less than the maintenance service fee for a car.

Fees and charges

The fees primary care physicians charge are less than what you or your insurance company will pay for a specialist. The annual compensation data for 2004 estimated that pediatricians, internists or family practitioners earn 50% of the annual income of a non- invasive cardiologist or a surgeon. I recently read an opinion about specialty choice trends among current medical students in which the comment was made that those who picked primary care as a specialty of choice were either naïve or foreigners. A primary care physician tends to order less expensive investigations in general and likely prescribes less expensive medications. She is well trained to handle at least 90% of all your health care needs even if you have a chronic illness. The key is to get the one PCP who is most suitable for you and your health condition.

Fringe benefits

She is also your health library key holder. Even with all the self-help books, it is easy to get lost in the vast ocean of medical science. Although the knowledge base is massive, it can look deceivingly simple.

Some may think that you see your PCP for annual check ups and go to the emergency room when you are sick. Yet I came across a web page offering corporate executives a comprehensive physical exam at one of the most prestigious hospitals in the nation, with a footnote, "This physical exam *will not* replace your primary care physician."

Almost all the specialists I know of now will ask you if you have a primary care physician with whom they can communicate. Why? Each specialist wants to do his job, looking after the area he is trained best to care for, but needs to report to the one doctor who looks at the big picture, your primary care provider. We are living in a highly specialized century in which each professional can excel only if he focuses on his specialty. You can compare your primary care physician to the general contractor who has to deal with the electrician, plumber, carpenter and other professionals to take care of your house.

The primary care physician, or as the HMO likes to call her, the gatekeeper, has another resource that adds value to the deal: inside information about the network of specialists that you or one of your loved one may need once in a while. To give you an idea, I do refer my patients to more than one dermatologist, as I've learned from my patients' feedback who is better than whom in treating acne or resistant warts. The same is true with any other specialty and subspecialty. As a primary care physician, I have the privilege of listening to plenty of real, untainted feedback about specialists in my network of physicians.

Long before the HMO started building structured and formal networks of physicians, your local primary care physician had already formed them. In the past, the primary care physician by design was considered the center of the physicians' nebulas, as all specialists in town had to be connected to their local primary care physicians to get the business. So even if you believe your primary care physician will not be able to solve your problem, I bet she will know better than anyone else who is the best qualified specialist physician to help you.

Your PCP will keep a complete record of your visits, referrals, immunizations, and medications in a personalized chart with your name on it. She must keep it protected and safe for years even if you relocate to another place. The information included in the chart can only be revealed with your permission, which means your wife or sister can't access it. If you get injured while playing baseball or soccer and the emergency room needs to know the date of your last tetanus shot, your record will have that information, so just contact your PCP's office.

It may not be possible every time, but if your primary care physician is familiar with your health, she may be able to help you even if you are out of town. One of my regular patients called me from California while vacationing to tell me her complaints. Because I knew her very well, I called in the medicines she needed. She felt better and saved quite a bit of time and money not going to an emergency room.

Want to know if the medication you use every day is getting pulled off the market because of a health risk? Your PCP's office gets updated warnings from the FDA and CDC.

A lot of my patients whom I send from time to time to a specialist for consultation or treatment come back to me and ask what specialist's report said. Many feel I am more down-to-earth than the specialist, while others just want to see if I agree. I read the report and translate it into plain English so that they can digest it better. Many want me to take over the treatment after the specialist's evaluation. Take ADHD kids for example: even for those needing psychiatric evaluation and support, once they're stabilized on a regular medication, I end up managing them for years. As I can also treat other conditions such as seizure disorders, cerebral palsy, chronic eczema, heart lesions and the like, some may only need to go back to the specialist once a year, or even less.

Despite all the benefits a PCP can provide, I believe that even with the introduction of HMO rules mandating a primary care provider for each member, the health care industry is still not utilizing that group of physicians properly. That is another reason for you the consumer to learn how to get more benefit from your primary physician.

When Should You Visit?

Some people have a condition called "Iatrophobia," or fear of doctors. Unfortunately this fear can prevent them from taking good care of their bodies.

I admit that I also delay my visits to my primary care doctor as much as I can, but procrastination is not a good idea. Healthy young people think their name is sealed somewhere on an immortality contract. But even if you owned the Fountain of Youth and drank from it every day, your body still needs maintenance to check organs and calibrate systems. It doesn't run forever on just food and water. Your body's organs and systems change constantly, and although sometimes you can feel the change yourself, other times you need someone to alert you before the changes harm you.

Young men and immortality

Young men are the most resistant group against buying into that concept as they only get a physical if they need it to play sports, enter school, or get a job. It is so manly to go to the gym or spend a whole day in a football game, but for a young man to see his doctor is not manly. My friends in psychology think that as males assume their masculine role in society, going to the doctor is perceived as a weakness when the masculine role demands strength. Yet this same young man who doesn't believe in annual check ups will never miss a 3-month oil change for his car.

Compiled statistics show that three visits to the doctor per year per person is the average. However, a breakdown of that data usually will reveal that some people visit the doctor a lot more than three times, while many do not see their doctor for years.

One of my patient's mothers was complaining about her husband who wants to make a record of how many years he has not seen a doctor. When she told me that she knew his cholesterol was high because it runs in the family, I didn't know what to say. Some believe if something isn't broken, don't fix it. While many people feel healthier if they don't go to see a doctor; I hope you're not one of them. The good news is that your primary care physician is the only doctor you need to visit if you're healthy and there is nothing wrong with you.

As you can tell from the national statistics, most of these three visits per year (more than 70%) were due to either acute or chronic illness. However, logic will suggest that if you visit the doctor on your own terms, you will get better results. When illness or injury is forcing that visit, the odds are that you just want to get it over with. You will spend the least time possible preparing for that visit, let alone having reasonable expectations.

Therefore, a good policy is to visit the doctor on your own terms once a year after you have done your homework.

But there are those who require more visits to the doctor than the average person. The term used in health care is *chronic illness*, such as diabetes, asthma, cerebral palsy, and many others. Let me introduce you to my frequent flyer program.

Frequent Flyers

Years ago while working in a high-risk pediatric clinic, one of my patient's mother said apologetically, "I'm sorry we have to come here so often." I smiled and told her not to worry about it, as I was enrolling her child in my frequent flyer program. As she seemed to feel much more at ease from that point on. I started using the term more often to let the mothers of my chronically ill children know that I value their visits. In all honesty, I believe the lessons I learned from those visits were much more valuable to me than my paycheck. Being part of a complex real human drama filled with moments of pain and agony, hours of anxiety, and days of victory and relief is an unparalleled experience.

What if you are a frequent flyer, in that you or your loved one needs to see your doctor more than 3 - 7 times per year? It is imperative you feel quite at ease in the doctor's office, as you would in your neighborhood café. Because you need to go to these visits more often than others, you should have the advantage of the Frequent Flyer program. Just as airlines offer perks and special treatment for their frequent flyers, you should enjoy those benefits too.

You should be acquainted with the receptionist, the medical assistant and the doctor, who should all know you well. You should be familiar with how the office works, including the best times to get in and out quickly. Your expectations should be higher than other customers; just like it would be of the service you get from the airlines if you are in one of their frequent flyer programs.

One mother smiled at me yesterday as she was telling me that she is signing up for the frequent flyer club because she is bringing her toddler so often to the clinic. She said, "You know we are going to get an RV and park right outside your clinic here." Another one said she wants to rent one of the exam rooms for her kids.

The frequent flyer program may include FREE services every now and then that may not be offered to other customers, such as samples of expensive medications, extra time with your provider, or maybe even a birthday gift.

The important thing is that it should not be a burden for you to go and see your doctor. If it is, you need to think about alternatives as you should not worry about getting your health care needs met when you have a chronic condition.

Why Do You Get Less?

Many of you may have never asked that question, or maybe you have no firm expectation for your doctor to live up to. When you go to a restaurant you have certain expectations about how long to wait for the food, quality of service, taste of the food, etc. You also want to compile some reasonable, measurable expectations for your doctor's visit that at least in your mind will determine how well the visit goes. I ask myself that question every day from my perspective as the primary care provider, but occasionally I ask it as a patient as well.

For example, one day I had a bad intestinal obstruction and knew I would be ending up admitted to the same hospital to which I admit patients. I made my rounds early in the morning, took care of my patients, then went straight down to the hospital emergency room to be admitted for my intestinal obstruction. In one morning I was both a doctor and a patient.

The following day, when my expectations of my surgeon were not met. I discharged myself against medical advice. (Don't do this unless you are a medical doctor.) However, I knew I was not getting from my surgeon the care and understanding I expected.

Even though I was sick as a dog when I was admitted, I had certain expectations I was not willing to compromise, including those for thoughtful care and two-way communication. As I improved, I tried to communicate better with my attending surgeon, but it was a lost battle. Fortunately my primary care physician was on my side, and that was enough for me. So at 6 PM after trying for two hours to reason with my surgeon, I asked for AMA (against medical advice) forms to sign and walked out.

My primary care physician agreed with me on getting a second opinion from another surgeon, a plan of care was set in motion, and the problem was solved. I assure you, I saved my health insurance company no less than $10,000 by doing what I firmly believed was the right thing. If we all do better jobs as consumers of health care, there's no doubt in my mind that the future will be better.

Let's try to be systematic and review the potential mistakes that may lead to your receiving less instead of more:

Three errors

The first error is the one you make before you go to the doctor, if you don't prepare well for that visit. The second is missing the opportunity to maximize your benefit from the visit while you are physically there, while the third is inadequate follow up to the visit.

In my opinion, anyone can get better results from a doctor's visit. By the end of this book, you should be able to:

1- Choose a doctor you are likely to trust
2- Prepare well for the visit.
3- Know what to expect.
4- Be there, body and mind during the visit.
5- Know how to use interactive communication during your visit.
6- Review the results of the visit and appreciate the follow-up process.

CHAPTER TWO
Sick or Well

Before we talk about how to research to get a good primary care physician, you need to ask yourself a simple question: why am I going? Physicians are trained to help you feel and get better when you are sick, or prevent you from getting sick. Simple enough— your visit is either to treat an illness (a sick visit) or to prevent one (a well visit.)

The illness can be one of two conditions, either acute (chest pain, sore throat) or chronic (asthma, diabetes.) What people label as a *follow-up visit* is really a focused sick visit for a specific ailment. When you use that term, it implies your diagnosis is known, so the visit will be short and limited to certain care items. Therefore I don't recommend you use the term *follow-up visit* if you're going to an office for the first time, as the receptionist may assume that you have been in the office before so you end up getting squeezed in between established patients.

Some patients will combine two types of sick visits in one, as a diabetic patient (chronic illness) can visit for chest pain (acute illness.) Or someone may combine a preventive visit with a chronic condition, such as a diabetic patient getting a physical exam and immunization. To simplify, remember the following line:

Preventive/Well   Sick (Acute)   Sick (Chronic)

Some will save time and money when they happen to be sick and it is time for their annual check up anyway, so they can hit two birds with one stone. Get your physical along with a prescription for your sore throat or sinus infection. The one who may save the most is a patient with a chronic illness (diabetes or asthma) who happens to have an acute illness (sinus infection) while he is scheduled for his annual physical exam. This patient will combine all three types of visits in one, a real combo deal if you ask me. If you're in a rush to find a doctor but your condition is not life-threatening (e.g. it doesn't involve bleeding, severe pain, difficulty breathing, etc.), remember that primary care physicians charge less than urgent care clinics just as urgent care clinics charge less than emergency rooms. Also remember that emergency room staff is not obligated to take care of chronic illness needs such as medication refills, and they may or may not stock immunizations. A few times I have patients who have gone to the emergency room for an outdoor injury for which they need a tetanus shot as their last one was more than five years before. However, because the ER had no tetanus shots, the patients had to come to my office the following day. They ended up with two visits and two different charges for one problem.

Another question you need to ask is: what are my expectations?

Expectations

As their family was being transferred to another city, the mother of one my patients asked what she should expect from the new doctor she would see. My answer was that doctors share the same technical knowledge from similar resources such as medical school education, residency training, board exams, textbooks, and professional journals, but each differs in his or her own professional experience. This professional experience gives each one of us a special flavor; some patients may love that particular flavor, and some may not. The meat is the same—it is just how you cook it, flavor it, dress it up, and of course present it. But at the end, the flavor shouldn't _harm_ any one of our patients. You know what Hippocrates said: if a physician can do no good, he should at least do no harm.

When you set your expectations, bet on professionalism rather than altruism. There are both overall general expectations and specific ones. General expectations include convenient location, accessible hours of operation, clean office, apparent compliance with health care standards of operations, and respectful and helpful staff. Above all, you expect a physician with whom you can communicate as well as trust.

What should you expect from your preventive visit?

1- You have been given the chance to inform your doctor of all your health data, including medical, mental, social, etc.

2- You have been given the chance to voice your health concerns to your doctor.

3- Your doctor has checked your body systems to your satisfaction.

4- You have been given a summary report about your physical condition.

5- You have received guidance on how to remain healthy.

6- You are satisfied with the treatment and care you experienced from the doctor and her office staff.

From your sick visit to the doctor you should expect:

1- Your doctor listened to your complaint or concerns.

2- Your doctor seems to understand why you are in her office today and not yesterday or next week.

3- You have been examined based on your complaint.

4- Your doctor took the time to tell you what is wrong and how she is going to help you feel better.

5- You feel that you understood all the instructions and recommendations given to you, from medication to investigation to follow-up plan or referral if needed.

What if your expectations are not met? Well keep reading this book you may find away.

Now that we have reasonable expectations to work with it is time to prepare.

Preparation Step One:

Research and Variables.

Now that you are motivated to see your primary care physician, the first step should be to find the one whom you are likely to get the most benefit out of visiting. The one you are more likely to keep. If you are looking for the best product in the market, what do you do? Search and *re*-search.

To organize your research for your perfect PCP, you need to think through the variables that will influence your choice. As in any research project, you need to identify your variables for a good outcome. Each of these variables will have an impact on your choice to a certain degree, but some may play a more important role than others based on your individual circumstances. I will try to shed some light on each of the variables; however, you will be the one who needs to calculate them based on how much influence each variable has on your choice. As each individual is different you may want to assign a value to each variable, say from 1 - 5. This will enable you to make better decisions for yourself.

1- **Medical insurance.** As I mentioned earlier, the basic three types of health insurance you will find in the market today are Traditional/FFS, HMO, and PPO.

The traditional kind is very flexible but tricky, as you have to know if office visits are covered, and if so, whether your plan covers wellness check ups and immunizations. Does it have a limit on how many visits per year, or on how much of the office visit charge is your responsibility?

By definition, HMOs must cover wellness check ups and immunizations because this is the whole philosophy behind their name (an ounce of prevention...) As a reminder, once you sign up with an HMO you are obligated to use their physician directory for your primary care physician or they may assign you one. The rule is necessary because you will not be able to go to any specialist unless your primary care doctor formally refers you (in writing.) You think everyone would know this by now, but think again. After decades of HMOs, I still have members of an HMO that forget that clause. On the other hand, a couple of the HMOs got smarter: they tell their members "you do not need a referral," but when it comes to a specialist recommendation, the primary physician has to approve any procedure. In general you tend to save more money with this arrangement.

If you are member of a PPO health insurance plan, you can combine decent savings and better choices. The PPO will provide you with a directory just like the HMO; if you find what you like, fine—you will be asked to pay less for visiting those doctors in the directory, so just keep the savings. Otherwise although the insurance will cover some or most, the PPO will ask you to pay more out-of-pocket for your encounter with an out-of-network physician.

If you are one of the tens of millions who are not covered by health insurance, the choice is yours to pick the primary care provider who suits your needs. The cost of services provided by primary care physicians is less than most medical services by hospitals, emergency rooms, or urgent care, as one of the worst and most expensive flaws in health care is utilizing the emergency room staff as primary care staff.

Let me give you a real life episode involving one of my patients who went to an urgent care facility for a fever and rash. His mom was told he had scarlet fever, given a prescription, and sent home. She called me on Sunday morning two days after he started the medication, complaining that he was not getting better. Because I hadn't seen him in months, I told her I couldn't give advice over the phone since fever and a rash in a child make up for a tricky list of diseases.

A phone diagnosis in a situation like this is treacherous. She reported the urgent care had told her that even though the child was seen fewer than two days ago in their place, she still had to bring him in and pay another set of charges because the doctors were not the same. Same illness, two visits, two charges.

This situation develops because in urgent care and emergency rooms, multiple physicians have to work to cover the extended hours of service. By health care industry standards, none of them is required to act as a personal physician for the patients they examine in the emergency room. As a matter of fact, sooner or later they are all required to notify your primary care physician of the reason for your visit. I get these reports every day although most of my patients have learned the proper way of using emergency rooms for fractures, breathing difficulties and the like.

But a few are not as yet with the program. I'm now looking at a long dictation from my colleague in the emergency room detailing a visit for no more than a simple virus. I skip to the end of third page of dictation to see what life-saving measure was taken, but find absolutely nothing. (Well, sometimes the patient may get an over-the-counter fever reducer.) On top of this, they instruct the patient to follow up with the primary care physician in 1 - 2 days. In summary, you end up having two physician visits for one sore throat, so you do the math.

Moneywise what you need to take into account when you have no insurance is that even though each clinical encounter is different, you can get very close to the actual charge if you tell the office your needs. The charges are based on the length of time the doctor spends with you and the type of procedures you need. Therefore you may save if you ask for a physical that doesn't include a hearing or vision screen. If you just had a chest X-ray done a few days ago and you are going in because of a cough, another chest X-ray may not be needed. If in doubt, ask how much the procedure will cost, as some may turn out to be a bargain if done in the primary care setting. Likewise, if you have a wart to be removed, the cost is likely to be less if done by a primary care provider than by a dermatologist.

In general most physicians' fees are tied to Medicare fees, which is information you can access from web sites on the Internet. Many physicians also sign discounted contracts with insurance companies to get their business. If you have no insurance but like your doctor, try to negotiate a deal with the office manager.

Some people think if they go to the county hospital or downtown emergency room, the health services are free; however, the truth is otherwise. All hospitals nowadays are quite serious about collecting all charges for each patient care as the subsidy from taxpayers can no longer sustain lax collection policies. Poor utilization of downtown emergency rooms burdened most county hospitals financial sheets with losses, so some have hired tough collection agencies to go after bad debts.

2- **You**. Age, sex, health condition and needs. YOUR personal preferences and past experiences. You don't have to be honest with anyone but yourself. If you are going to expose your body and mind to someone whom you are unwilling to trust, you are asking for less than what you deserve.

Primary care physicians come in all colors, styles and shapes, as they are a more diverse group of doctors than you think. As I mentioned before, because most primary care residency programs know that those are the doctors who make the least money, they accept a lot more minorities and foreign medical graduates than any specialized residency program. I was there—I know.

While in training at Children's hospital in Detroit, Michigan, I met ONE pediatric neurosurgeon who was female *and* African American. Yet I've seen tens of female African-American pediatricians, family physicians and internists. You want to validate my statement in general, look at the physician and surgeon section in your local Yellow Pages, or better yet open up your local hospital web site and browse under medical staff directory. Search the hospital medical staff first for primary care physician names, and then search the staff directory for plastic surgeon names. Then you will know exactly what I mean.

Recently I was chatting over dinner with one of my old clinical instructors from a children's hospital who had been working there since he graduated from his hometown medical school in India. I asked why the hospital board hadn't awarded the chairmanship position (the highest clinical post) to one of the two renowned department chiefs who had served the hospital for decades. He replied they only give those positions to certain people, as skin color makes a difference. I understand this was his own perception of the process, but not necessarily the truth.

Does gender or race influence patients' perception of the doctor? Many have researched that subject and found some interesting results.

First, researchers KA.Hunt and A.Gaba on perception of health care by minorities concluded that racial and ethnic minorities are more likely than whites to have lower levels of trust or satisfaction with their physician. Disparate levels of trust and satisfaction exist within ethnic and minority populations, even when controlling for the distribution of individuals across types of health plans.

D.A.Barr from the Department of Sociology at Stanford University conducted a study of the relationship between race/ethnicity and patient satisfaction. The results showed that when a 4-item, physician-specific scale was used, *nonwhite patients were less satisfied than white patients with their direct interaction with the physicians included in the study.*

Your perception of reality is your reality and to select a physician you need to work with your reality. Physicians take a professional oath to be fair, just and nondiscriminatory, but you don't. You're the one who benefits the most from trusting your physician. If you have a problem with gender, race, or ethnic group, you should search for the doctor you are likely to trust with the characteristics you want. If for whatever reason you can't do that, at least choose the one you distrust the least. (I'm told many voters do that every four years in presidential elections.)

3-   **Location.** With some exceptions, most of us will be able to pick a primary care physician within a 10-mile radius from home. Physician distribution statistics in 2004 noted a variation in the availability of primary care physicians based on location. The national average of the number of patients per one primary care physician is 1321. If you are one of the 62 million or so Americans who live in a county outside a metropolitan statistical area (i.e., a less populated area), the ratio of patients per primary care physician changes to 1810 patients per primary care physician. So on average you may have a third less options to find your personal doctor.

On the other hand you are more likely to be satisfied with your doctor. Donahue and E. Ashkin from the Department of Family Medicine at the University of North Carolina, Chapel Hill studied rural population's satisfaction with their physicians. Their conclusion was that over half of the rural population studied had seen the same physician for more than five years. Longer continuity of care was associated with greater patient satisfaction and confidence in one's physician, but not with a greater likelihood of receiving recommended preventive services.

4- **Resources available to you for your research.** The best tool in this day and age is Internet access. The abundance of information you get from the Internet is likely more than you will ever need. The other important resource is your personal ties with friends, neighbors or co-workers.

In addition to official reports about doctors from web sites, you need some human feedback to help your research. The combination of the web and a friend is as close as you can get to perfection.

No, I didn't forget what they write in health magazines and articles about calling your hospital referral department or local medical society—if you have no Internet access, go right ahead and use the phone. But cruising the Internet at home or in your library will provide you with a wealth of information in record time. Some information can be redundant or too much, but you will decide what to review and what to ignore. A good wed site to locate physicians is WebMD.

http://doctor.webmd.com/physician_finder/home.
aspx?sponsor=core

5- Time.

If you know what you want and have Internet access, it should take you less than an hour to come up with a list of primary care physicians near you to choose from. You don't want or need to spend too much more time than necessary doing your research. Serendipity, a phenomenon of finding valuable or agreeable things not sought for, is a fringe benefit of research. You will learn in a few minutes of research both terms and facts about health care that you would not have known otherwise.

A list of 3 - 5 physicians is a reasonable one to work with in most cases. You want to keep that list for some time in case later your first choice does not satisfy your expectations. Even with good preparation, there is nothing more real than face-to-face interaction between you and your primary care physician, so that's the best way to make your final choice.

Now, if you have a directory from a **PPO** or **HMO** health plan, look under the primary care providers list, as almost every doctor now has a web page (whether he knows about it or not.) You can cruise doctors' web pages to obtain background information, office hours, and areas of professional interest in addition to general medical practice, etc.

If you don't have any of the above, look at your Yellow Pages' directory on the web. As you aren't limited to those in a directory from a health plan company, you have more choices, but you need to go to your state medical licensing board web site to make sure that whomever you're adding to your list carries a current medical practice license. You will be able to find more about the physician's credentials on the web, but just for the sake of time, wait until you have made a preliminary list to choose from.

Make your preliminary list of 3 - 5 names ready for a final run. But let's stop here for a quick review:

Review

Why am I going to the doctor?
Well/Preventive Visit Sick Visit

Do I have health insurance that covers office visits?
Yes   No

If No, skip the next question.

What type?

HMO   PPO   Traditional/POS

My preferences are.

Gender   Race   Other

The following doctors meet my criteria:

1-

2-

3-

4-

5-

Step Two in Preparation:

Narrowing Your Options and Choosing

You are confident now that your choice will be based on a good foundation. You learned about yourself (likes and dislikes) and the list of potential physicians from whom you will choose. I bet if you have spent time researching your choice of physician, you will walk into the office more open-minded, less intimidated and much at ease.

As we are talking about choices, let me share a line I heard thirty years ago. Someone was admiring the system in communist countries. Why? He said "having one choice is the easiest choice: you do not have to think too hard." But I sure hope that here and now, no one still thinks that way. I understand if you're in prison, you may have no choice, but if you're free, you should have options from which to select.

Now let's open the doors for physician profiling. If you don't have access to the Internet, I'm sorry but you must get access now. Then all you do is type those two words (*physician profile*) on the search engine, get to your area of interest and specific names of doctors, and search name by name down the list. A word of caution though: the last time I typed in my name, it resulted in 147 web sites, only a few of which gave good information about credentials, practice location, office hours and the like although these data make up a good physician profile. It's not that hard to determine which web sites are more valuable: those would be the hospital, health insurance, state board of medicine and American Medical Association sites. For the sake of time, collect the basic information that matters to you the most and set it up so you can compare the physicians on your list. I know you will be tempted by information that's interesting but means nothing to your search, but stay focused, as otherwise you will get lost in this process.

Details that matter to you are:
1- Credentials: medical education, internship and residency training, board certification, state medical license and Drug Enforcement Agency (DEA) license.
2- Specific areas of clinical interest in addition to general medical practice.
3- Current malpractice insurance.
4- Hospital affiliation.
5- Participation in health insurance (the one you have.)
6- Office hours and general policies. How long is the wait for a Well visit and how long for a Sick visit? Can weekend and late hours be used for non-urgent visits?

If surfing the Internet frustrates you, call each office and ask the above questions. It will be more scientific if you compare answers in a grid-like format, which may also save you time. If you want be methodical and give each physician/practice a score and grade from top to bottom, go ahead. Remember to keep this score for a year just in case you or another family member wants to review it. At the end, pick your best bet, the one your research suggests can give you the most benefit. The one you are likely to TRUST. You have done all of the above to get to that trust process by first verifying credentials, reviewing background information, and validating what your friends have told you about the doctor.

Step Three in Preparation:

Act

1- Call **for an appointment**. When you call the doctor's office for an appointment, the question you'll be asked is simple: why do you want to see the doctor?

Every doctor's office divides visits into "urgent" and "can wait" kinds of appointments. Before you make the call, you have to make that decision for yourself so as to be persuasive on the other end. For most people, regular physical exams are not urgent, unless you need it soon for a job offer or your son is going to football practice tomorrow. In these situations, use your skills of negotiations to be convincing. Try to explain to the receptionist the urgency of your situation, and if all else fails, ask to speak to the office manager or even your chosen doctor, as one of them should be able to break the rules for you.

Years ago I worked in a very busy children's clinic where the day after school started, the phone didn't ever stop ringing as parents were asking for urgent appointments for a school physical. We tried for years to get the message to parents to do the physicals in the summer time, as they would still be acceptable to any school board, but our efforts were in vain. It was simply impossible to get all these physicals done within the time frame parents felt appropriate. So parents got really creative, as they would call to reserve a Sick appointment; then as I examined the child in the room, the parents would hand me the school physical form to sign.

The one incident I will never forget is when a high school coach sent me a physical form checked with my signature on it, as he didn't think it was my true signature that he knew from other forms. He was right: the mother forged my signature on the form to allow her son to participate in school sports. I hope none of you would ever pull a trick like that. These are the kinds of risks that are not worth taking.

For an urgent matter, most people can get into their doctor's office on the same day they call. If you are being denied a same-day visit and you know for sure you need to be seen, you should let the office manager know that you are unsatisfied with the situation and want her to talk to the doctor. You should also tell her that if the matter can't be resolved, you may switch to another doctor. However, remember that abusing this rule may force you to change from one primary care physician to another. Switching for good reasons is fine, but if you keep on changing from one primary care provider to another year after year, you will not get the most benefit. If the office tells you that you are being squeezed in, they are letting you know that it may take longer than usual to get you in and out of the office, but it shows that they care and are willing to work with you to keep you satisfied.

The early bird and the lunch hour

The best time to call for an appointment is the first thing in the morning, as almost all the offices I've seen have more times available before noon than after noon. Most doctors I've worked with also perform better and are in a better mood during morning hours. The bottom line: by all means gets the morning appointments as often as you can. As an added bonus, if ever you need to go for a blood test, X-ray or even a referral to a specialist, they may be able to accommodate you in the same day, while that's not likely to happen if you don't visit your doctor until 4 or 5 PM.

To avoid traffic jams in the office, try to skip Mondays and Fridays. Another trick for making routine annual appointments such as your regular physical examination is to choose summer rather than wintertime. As from mid-May to Labor Day most offices experience a slowdown, if you choose a summer date, you are likely to wait less and have more of the doctor's time to ask any questions you have without being rushed.

Another tip: offices that don't start at 8 AM may work through the lunch hour or after 5 PM, which can be a way for you to avoid using your sick time from work for your appointment. Some will extend hours of operations beyond 5 PM once a week or so.

Schedule your day around the visit so you're not in a rush to leave before getting things done. In general, doctors are notorious for losing track of time during exciting clinical duties. One hospital administrator I remember used to have meeting after meeting to remind us about the cost of time: the impossible comparison between the way lawyers and accountants work around a perfect time frame and the inefficiency of our working day habits.

In real life, you can't guarantee that when you go to the office, there will be no sick patients that need more time than was previously budgeted, or that someone forgot his appointment all together. The upside is that the cancellation/no show rate in many medical offices is about 25% to 30%, so you may get lucky and spend less time in the office than you anticipated.

2- **Prepare the documents you need.** Your insurance card is important, but don't panic if you can't find it (Murphy's Law #1) because the physician's office can use an identification number to verify your insurance coverage over the phone or Internet. Remember health maintenance organization cardinal rule which states "if you are one of their members, *you must select a primary care physician or you will be assigned one*". You will not be able to visit another primary care physician unless you call and make the necessary changes.

Another important document is a copy of your own previous medical records or your child's immunization record. If you need special forms from your employer or school filled out, place them in one folder for easy access. I can't tell you how many times parents realize as they're leaving the exam room that they forgot to bring the documents for me to sign. That means you have to waste more time going back to find them, then mail or even bring them back in. Mark my words, I bet you in the near future some smart guy will make all this happen over the Internet, but for now be sure you have the documents with you.

As a rule, use your medical chart as a safe deposit box for clinical documents by asking the office staff to keep a copy of your pertinent documents in the chart, even if procedures were done somewhere else.

At the beginning of every school year, my office receives many calls from parents, schools, and day care centers asking for immunization records to be faxed. I wish I could tell that you'll never lose your child's immunization card, but I can't, as most parents misplace those shot records sooner or later. But your friendly primary care provider staff can keep a copy in the chart as your medical safe deposit box.

I really appreciated what one of the mothers did who joined my clinic after coming from a different state. Two weeks before her children's appointment, she stopped by the office and handed me personally copies of her three children's medical records. This gave me enough time to study the records so as to cut down on the time she needed to spend telling me their history. And now the old records are also part of the new medical chart.

3- **Gather your personal health concerns; collect your thoughts** (even better in writing.) The information you hand to your doctor is very important to the success of your visit. On many occasions, I get parents that each subsequent visit keep adding to the family history information they hadn't mentioned before. One couple finally remembered to tell me they both had a strong family history of asthma only after the third time in six weeks their infant came into the office wheezing and coughing. That piece of information changed their childcare plan. I will elaborate on this subject next.

History

That brings me to the subject of HISTORY. Not the history you studied in school—we're talking about your medical history. A good medical history should be truthful, complete and concise.

In medical textbooks, the history component of the clinical encounter is so important that medical students are grilled on the art of taking it. A correct medical diagnosis without good medical history can be time consuming, expensive and risky. What questions to ask for what symptom or concern? It is the first of four parts that your doctor will document on your visit clinical notes. It is entirely your responsibility, as what you say will prompt what your doctor will do. Believe me, if you do a good job understanding and summarizing your history, you will get the best return on every minute you spend preparing your medical history.

When I introduce the clinical encounter documentation you shall notice that medical history is the first of four components.

History for this purpose is broken down into subcategories ranging from demographic to social, environmental, etc. (about 13 to 15 in all), some of which are mandatory for every visit, and some which are specific for certain situations or age groups. For example, pediatricians like to dwell on developmental history and immunizations while obstetricians are likely to zoom onto menstrual and birth history.

While teaching medical students and pediatric residents at MSU Flint/Hurley campus, I used to say that if it takes you less than two hours and five pages to get the patient's history, your history documentation is not complete. For the most part it did take them about that long.

Before the age of MRI and ultrasound, doctors used to listen to the patient's history carefully, and some still do now. Well executed and communicate medical history can lead to an accurate diagnosis as experience taught me. To insure that you get the best possible care, do your part by learning how to efficiently summarize your medical history.

Let me start by listing the medical history components from the doctor's point-of-view:

1- **Chief complaint** (abbreviated version of why you are visiting your doctor.) think of this as your punch line.

2- **History of the present illness:**
History of the chief complaint or history of present illness (detailed version of your complaint.) If you are sick, talk about the onset and location of your complaint (i.e., left or right.) Also mention the duration (how long you've been suffering) and character (specify the type of pain or describe it.) Be sure to mention aggravating and associated factors (e.g. what makes the pain worse, or that you also suffer from dizziness with your headache.) Relieving factors are the opposite but also important: those are what make the pain less. It will also help if you can

grade your pain or headache on a scale from 1 - 10, or at least as being mild, moderate or severe.

3-   **Review of systems**. In this section your doctor will ask you about symptoms you didn't mention when you started (i.e., do you have any other problems?) Some doctors will systematically list potential problems in relation to different body systems or organs with the intent being to obtain a complete picture of the person coming in for the visit, but this may or may not give clues to the problem. I use this part occasionally to validate a vague or no specific complaint. When I get a healthy looking school age child, I ask, "in addition to the stomach ache that made you skip school today, does your head hurt? Do you feel weak? Do you have a problem seeing or moving?" Many fall into the trap and start complaining about more symptoms which can only be associated together if someone is faking an illness. Doctors don't have any lie detectors, but they do have a lot of knowledge and experience, so if you want to deceive your doctor, do a lot of reading.

3-   **Past medical history**. In a nutshell, this covers any major health problem you've endured, including hospitalization, surgery, accident or injury. If you have only a brief summary, that fine's to say it orally, but if your past medical history is extensive, I urge you to write it down or bring a copy of previous medical records. There may have been tests and investigations that may or may not need to be repeated, immunizations that need to be updated, or medications that need to be refilled.

4- **Allergies**. About 20% of the patients I see in my practice are allergic to one thing or another: environment, mold, cold, food items, or medications. Allergic reactions to medications happen at such a distressing frequency that every encounter document in every medical chart has an entry for allergies. Because reactions are preventable, everyone has to help out, including you who have the most important task of knowing your allergies well and always reminding everyone in the office about them. They should also be documented on your medical chart, but sometimes even that may not be sufficient, as the information may be virtually hidden or you may be dealing with an alternate covering physician. I have many patients who every time I write them an antibiotic prescription, ask me: does it have penicillin? This a good habit and an excellent reminder to whomever is taking care of you so as to avoid mishaps.

5- Medications. What are the medications you are now using? Start with prescription medicines, but don't forget the over-the-counter ones. You must have noticed by now how many medications are listed as over-the-counter, with that list expanding daily. While helping to relieve your symptoms, many of these medications can also negatively affect you. In particular, over-the-counter medications can interact with your prescription medication, with some of these interactions being serious or even fatal.

6- **Family history.** Most people think of their immediate family (parents, brothers and sisters), but in medicine family history branches out as far as the DNA can go. The genetic pieces that put us together extend back to Adam and Eve. Of particular importance are the people in your family tree who were diagnosed with known inheritable diseases such as diabetes, asthma, muscular dystrophy, psoriasis, breast cancer, etc.

7- **Social history.** It sounds like an invasion of privacy, but this gives your caregiver a chance to know more about your situation, limitations and risk factors. When we used to give an oral polio vaccine, I had to ask about the possibility of exposing a living relative who might be immunosuppressed (i.e. someone with AIDS, being treated for cancer, or on a high dose of steroids.) This question was necessary because a child may pass along components of the vaccine that could endanger those are immunosuppressed. Other social factors can affect treatment. For example, I had a very long discussion with a divorced mother who wanted me to prescribe ADHD medication for her 8-year-old. However, as the child's father didn't believe in medication, he wouldn't administer the medication to the child on the days he had custody. Therefore the odds were against the therapy being successful because the medication only works if given daily.

8- **Psychological history.** Tell your doctor if you have been diagnosed with a psychological disorder such as depression, or if you feel unusual or strange feelings. Most people think pediatricians handle psychological disorders or mental problems of children. I honestly think that we as pediatrician see the vast majority of post partum depression in women. Post partum depression is fairly common among women after delivery, and most of the time it is quite mild. Most new mothers talk to me about occasional sad feeling and occasional crying. What I was not prepared for was the sever form, I was not trained to handle those. A couple of years after my graduation. I met a very nice, highly educated couple planning to have their first child. I felt they are both ready and mature for the task, they will make a perfect parent team. Shortly after the delivery, I noted the mother having more emotional labiality than I have seen before, especially that the baby is in perfect condition. She was coming with baby to the clinic a lot more than what was needed for his regular care, and I was not sure what was going on. Finally I got a call from her husband that she became so hyper, could not control her train of thoughts and had to be admitted to the psychiatric ward for inpatient management. I learned form other cases that post part depression can be progress to a sever form, it can also flare up underlying psychological disorders. What I found from my practice is that so many people are ashamed of psychological disorders. No one hesitates to discuss an episode of pneumonia, or bad stomach problem. When it comes to depression or bipolar disorders many feel guilty enough that they would rather omit that history. For the example I mentioned earlier, both parents confined to me later that the mother and her family did have a history of bipolar disorder.

If you don't feel guilty when fall ill with influenza why would you feel guilty if suffer from depression or anxiety?

9- **Environmental history.** Exposure to cigarette smoking is number one on this list, whether you yourself smoke or you're exposed to someone else who does. Other exposures are also important. I ask about lead because many children are at risk of lead poisoning, as the paint used inside homes for years contained it; exposure to high levels presents a serious health risk. Others to keep in mind are mercury and carbon monoxide.

10- **Developmental history.** I am interested in the child's development including speech, motor and sensory skills and social skills, as these bits of information are critical for pediatricians. When I ask the question "so how the baby's development?" to some of the new mothers they mistake it for weight gain. Developmental miles stones are standardized expectations of what human achieve at specific age. From birth forward, each age brings new achievements. You will find these information in print in any pediatrician or family practice office, a good web site to find developmental milestones is www.kidsgrowth.com. As a parent you owe to your child to monitor their development, and pick unexpected delays in achievement to discuss it with his primary care physician. Unfortunately many children with a range of developmental problems can be missed if their history is revealed and discussed in the right time. Disorders such as autism, speech delay or hearing disorders can be managed sooner if the diagnosis is made on time.

11- **Immunization history.** This particular information is gaining a lot more attention from the Bird Flu scare to the annual flu vaccination. When taking your child to her pediatrician, always carry her immunization card. Not only may the staff ask you about previous vaccinations, but also we have been adding so many new vaccinations to the list, your child is likely to need one sooner or later. As a reminder to adults, vaccines are not just for children we all need them. Tetanus vaccine every 5- 10 years is indicated for all. So is "Hepatitis B vaccine" and "Flu" vaccine if you can get to it on time. Patients with chronic conditions such as diabetes, asthma, immune problem should regularly ask their primary care physician about updates to the vaccine list. In this part of the history you want to mention any major side effect to any vaccination.

12- **Menstrual.** I tell girls to keep a calendar as when they begin their cycle. The menstrual cycle can be irregular for a couple of years till ovulation begins. This irregularity "the period does not come at the same time every month" creates anxiety among many. Occasionally the menstrual cycle length differs from one female to another. The menstrual cycle is a critical marker for very complex hormonal and biological events taking place in your body.

13- **Nutritional.** What are your eating habits? Some people are vegetarians, while some just like added vitamins. Some have difficulty consuming milk while others drink too much. Some say you are what you eat, but I don't think so. But for those of us who suffer from diseases such as gout, diabetes, GERD (Gastroesophygeal reflux disease), and so many others, you need to talk to your primary care physician honestly about your eating habits as they will influence disease activity, severity, and needed care. It may influence the choice of medications being offered to treat health condition, or the result of a test. As I examine some of the infants or toddler, I notice the skin's yellow color but normal color eyes, and I would smile and say to the parents *are you feeding your child a lot of carrots?* I love the way the parents look so astonished and say *yah he loves carrots and sweet potato, how did you know?* Excessive intake of both leads to condition called "Carotenemia" which is usually harmless but causes the yellowish skin color. Carotenemia can be mistaken for a more serious condition called "Jaundice".

Having mentioned all these components of the medical history, you can imagine how much time and mental effort you are going to save be preparing these bites of data ahead of time.

Now that you are ready to go, how should you dress for the visit?

Dress code

There is absolutely no dress code; I have never seen any sign in a doctor's office that tells you what or what not to wear. But even though it is entirely up to your choice and taste, allow me to make some humble suggestions. As you're not going out on a date, you probably want to dress conservatively. However, a three-piece suit is not a good option for the doctor's visit unless you're going back to or coming from work. I've seen patients come in wearing fancy clothes which take quite a while to take off or put back on, so you don't need to do that. Be practical: sometimes you may need to give a blood sample or be sterilized with betadine, procedures that may stain your clothes even if done with care; the stain from either is tough to remove, and doctors are not known to pay for their patients' dry cleaning. Therefore choose a loose, comfortable, easy-to-clean outfit. If the outfit is loose enough, you may be spared the fashionable patient's gown (I can't promise you that, as I worked with a colleague who insisted that any patients coming for a physical exam must take off all their clothes and wear the official patient gown.)

But don't get too comfortable either. I've had many people come in their sleepwear. Some had a good reason to do so, but many could have easily changed before the visit.

For males who decline to wear underwear, I advise you to listen to those guys who have ended up in the emergency room because their penile foreskin was trapped in a zipper. Added bonus? They had to be triaged by a female nurse or medical assistant, and many times the emergency room doctor was also a female.

Smelling good is not required, but everyone in the office will appreciate your smelling clean. As most offices now are small with limited space, any strong smell will be quite noticeable. Smell also can tell your doctor about smoking or drinking habits you've forgotten to confess. When my wife worked with me in the office, she said it was a two-way street, so she kept reminding me about mints, mouthwash, and chewing gum.

Now we are done with the preparation, let me take you to the office.

CHAPTER THREE
Inside The Office

<u>Front Desk/front look</u>

Here, you are: you've found the place, parked your car, and opened the office door. Look for the front desk window where you will find a clipboard marked "sign in sheet." The person sitting right behind that window may be busy doing many other tasks at once, but now you are her responsibility. She may be alone if the practice is small or one of the front desk team if the practice is big. Let us talk about the front desk and see how we can utilize it better.

Even though most medical offices now use a staff who can perform multiple duties, you need to think of the staff as being two different professionals. When you enter the office, the nice lady sitting behind the glass window handing you the sign-in sheet probably has no medical or clinical training. Her duties are primarily administrative. The front desk personnel are there to take care of paperwork, answer the phone, attend to insurance matters, complete referral forms, manage computer software, send and receive faxes, prepare and sort medical records, and perform the many other administrative duties the office requires to function.

Despite this difference in duties, I've witnessed many people start talking to the front desk person about medical or clinical issues just because the person is wearing a nurse's outfit or white coat. They may ask whether their son is due for immunization or even what they should use for constipation. These are questions that should be asked when you are in the room with your physician. Alternatively, the medical assistant who will help you get to your exam room may also be able to answer some of your medical concerns or at least write them down for your doctor to answer.

Most of my clients are parents, many of whom establish an easy bond with the front desk staff. Often they insist on asking them medical questions, even after they have already seen me. These nice front desk ladies have to come back and relay the questions to me, then bring back the answer to the waiting parent. My guess is the front desk staff is the most visible, accessible and customer-friendly part of the office.

Therefore if you want to know something about billing, need a copy of your child's immunization record, or want to schedule a follow-up appointment, talk to the front desk lady. She will take care of your request very efficiently. But if you have a question about medication or a clinical issue, wait until you see your doctor or her medical assistant.

In most offices you will find the front desk receptionist is the easiest and most available person to talk to. Ask her about any information you may not have received before your visit: anything ranging from the doctor's credentials to his pager or emergency contact number, or to your insurance coverage limitations. If you are upset about the care you received or want to complain, ask for the office manager. Under HIPAA (Health Insurance Portability and Accountability Act) regulations, all medical offices have to integrate a customer complaint process into the office setting. The likely person to handle your complaint will be one of the front desk staff.

Now that you know about the front desk, let me seat you in the waiting room.

Waiting Room and the truck load

Medical offices try to make the waiting room as acceptable and agreeable to their patients as possible. Keep it clean and uncluttered, but have some magazines or maybe a TV (some can even afford to have cable channels and a plasma TV set.) To some doctors the waiting room is a statement. While affluent plastic surgeons may have expensive art pieces hanging on the walls, cushiony real leather seats, and gourmet coffee, I doubt my colleagues in primary care are going to be able to offer you such luxury, as they need to watch out for overhead expenses. As I've mentioned before, we primary care physicians are considered to be at the bottom of the food chain.

One of the frustrating problems that many patients complain about is the waiting time. I just read a piece in the February 13, 2005 *Detroit Free Press* written by author Mitch Albom (*The Five People You Meet in Heaven*) about waiting in his doctor's office for 47 minutes just to get his blood drawn..

The irritation caused by waiting has been studied by many health care organizations because it is an important complaint that had been echoed by patients for years. Because primary care providers handle so many urgent requests, many people probably put them at the top of the list, and despite quite a few discussions, proposals and suggestions, you can tell from the Albom article that this problem hasn't gone away.

But let me run some math equations by you. First, most experts will tell you that for a primary care physician to generate a full-time income, she will have to care for about 2000 patients, while others will say at least 1600 - 1800. Popular doctors will carry even more of a patient load in primary care. As the average number of visits per patients is three per year, your primary care physician needs to see between 30 to 40 patients per working day. Here is another difficulty: the "no show rate, " in which the percentage of patients who are on the schedule but don't show up for their appointment varies from 15 to 30%. So for the office manager to keep her job, she better allow 50 names to be on the schedule.

Oh, one more element: you have the right under the "unwritten policy" to be 15 - 20 minutes late for your appointment and still be seen. What really happen in the office is that the doctor may be sitting for an hour or so with no patients, then all of a sudden a truckload arrive. As in the restaurant business, if you want dinner at 6 PM on a Friday night, you're going to stand in line for a while.

In a restaurant, they will give you preference if you have a reservation, but in the doctor's office the sickest person has to go in first. It is very difficult in day-to-day scheduling to get everyone in and out as efficiently as many of us want. However, the front desk person should be helpful if you ask how long the wait will be, as she already knows how the day is going so far or if there's been a delay or cancellation. But even if you are a regular customer to the office, it's better to budget for extra waiting time.

I'm one of those people who hate waiting at all, let alone waiting to see a doctor who is likely to tell me things I don't enjoy hearing, such as to eat less fat or spicy food. Therefore I pick up a magazine I've never had the time to read before and try and indulge myself. When I used to take my daughter to her doctor, she provided her mom and me with all the entertainment we needed, as she grabbed toys to share with us and pointed to the many objects in the room that a 3-year-old found fascinating. We were constantly answering the questions she kept asking about a hanging picture, odd-looking chair, or colorful magazine. Because she is a very tactile person, she touched as many toys, table surfaces, and chair arms as she could. Watching her move and interact with a new environment was fun. She made the wait go by so fast I almost counted it as quality family time.

Some of my patients come with their books to read or homework to finish. Some use their cell phone, Game Boy or iPod as entertainment. Others socialize with whomever they meet in the waiting room. Very few use the time the so-called proper way: reading some of the updated health information scattered everywhere in the waiting room. I'm sure all consider this boring; honestly I don't read this material because I like to relax and collect my thoughts before I see my doctor. I also try to be as time efficient as humanly possible to avoid more visits. I admit I may not be as an exemplary patient as I should, but I think the best way to be less bored is to use the waiting time for activities that will likely to relax you.

Exceptions to the waiting rules exist; for example, if you or your child have a case of chicken pox or shingles, let the front desk know in private as we like to keep highly contagious conditions from spreading. This usually means you will get into a separate room as soon as possible. Also if you have a condition that impairs or weakens your immune system, let the staff know ahead of time as you do not want to contact germs while waiting in the doctor's office.

But to assure you, a clean, comfortable waiting room will be there for you. As an average waiting time of 30 minutes is reasonable, if you're in a rush ask the front desk staff about possible additional delay and she will explain to you the reason it may occur.

Hostility in the office

Many of the mothers who bring their kids to my office establish a nice friendly relationship with my front desk workers and office manager. I have to tell you that those mothers get many perks and have a very easy time getting in and out of the office. Even while you are sick or distressed, if you can, be courteous to the ladies upfront as they do want to make life better for you and your family.

The more hostile you are to the nice lady upfront, the less likely that you're going to get the best out of your visit. All medical insurance plans allow the doctor's office to Terminate/ Transfer care or discharge a patient who is discourteous or abusive to the staff. There are standard written procedures with which managers and administrators are familiar for handling these unfortunate circumstances. Here is an example of how this policy may state conduct that will be a cause for termination:

The patient or guardian exhibits violent or life threatening behavior involving physical acts of violence, physical or verbal threats of violence against a health care provider or provider's staff; threats or violence at a provider's location; or when the patient/ guardian is determined to be an excessive menace to a provider or provider's staff.

No one in the office likes to be involved in one of these episodes, but once in a while we have to go by the book. In a professional place like your doctor's office, public behavior is expected to be in accordance with general courtesy. There are many eyewitnesses in the waiting room in case of a dispute or disagreement. The last time I had to discharge one of my favorite patients because her divorcing parents brought their anger and hostility to each other to my waiting room. As the police had to become involved in this incident, you can imagine how difficult it would be for me to maintain professional objectivity.

Your Rights

On the other hand, it is your right to be treated fairly and with professional courtesy. If the front desk personnel treats you otherwise and you're not sure who is the office manager, make a point of talking to your doctor about your concerns even before he starts his clinical encounter. After all, he may wonder why you are in such an angry mood or why your heart rate and blood pressure are elevated.

This is an example of a patient's rights:

- *Receive quality health care.*
- *Be treated with respect.*
- *Consider care that safeguards your personal dignity and respects your personal values.*
- *Be seen by a personal doctor who will arrange the care you need.*
- *Get all the facts from your personal doctor about your health and treatment.*
- *Help make decisions about the health care you get.*
- *Say no to any medical treatment with which you disagree.*
- *Know the names and backgrounds of your health care providers.*
- *Get help with any special disability needs you may have.*
- *Get help with any special language needs you may have.*
- *Tell your personal doctor how you wish to be treated if you ever become too ill to decide yourself.*
- *Have your medical records kept confidential.*
- *Get a copy of your medical records.*
- *Voice your concern about the service or care you receive.*

If you want more details about your rights and

responsibilities, go to http://www.hcqualitycommission.gov/final/append_a.html.

Medical Chart or safe deposit box

While you are waiting, let me tell you what the front desk is doing: they are organizing your medical chart. This is the safe deposit box where your health records will be maintained and kept.

The health care industry is extremely regulated for obvious reasons, the most important being that it is all about life, death and the quality of life we live. One of the main requirements in the health care industry is the necessity of establishing medical records for each individual (patient) visiting the office. Each doctor's office must show a range of people from regulators from insurance companies to federal and stat authorities that they are competent in keeping and maintaining a medical record for each of the patients they encounter. The future trend is to eventually convert the paper format of the traditional medical records into the 21st century paperless Electronic Medical Records (EMR). It is believed this concept will improve quality and enhance efficiency in the health care field. Large and medium-size organizations are already amid the change, while small players are moving slowly and waiting for better deals, just like most people do for new products (compare the price of a 42-inch plasma TV in 2003 with 2006.)

However, the fundamentals are similar all over:

Location: your medical record (chart) is usually kept in the same office you visit if it is a small group of physicians. However, in large physician groups or hospital outpatient clinics, your medical record may be in another location called a medical records department or medical information department.

Contents: your medical record must have your identification data, including name, date of birth, gender, social security number, address, and telephone number. It usually also has a medical record number for better access and confidentiality. In addition, it should have your emergency contact telephone numbers (in case of a panic laboratory value or X-ray.) Your medical insurance information is usually updated once a year in the records.

In most cases, the medical chart is organized so as to open to a summary of your visits and list of medications you use. The summary page is sometimes called the problems list. Even though you may not have any problem, your chart must have that page. It also highlights any allergy you have, the last date you were in the office, and the investigations you have gone through.

The rest of the chart is divided into compartments that separate the doctor's notes from outside investigations, referrals, previous medical records, immunization records, flow charts and other pertinent documents needed for your health care.

Importance: your personal medical records are very valuable documents, but ones which I've noticed many people underutilize. They contain personal health data, including your weight and height, blood pressure, history of illness, medications you used, vaccinations you received, and a lot more. The medical chart records, maintains and accumulates important data about you year after year. Therefore if you move from place to place, keep a copy with you to be added to your new doctor's chart.

Legality: your medical records are also considered a legal document protected under many privacy rules. Congress passed the most recent a few years ago with HIPAA, short for HEALTH INSURANCE PORTABILITY AND ACCOUNTABILITY ACT. HIPAA rules are meant *to protect the use, transfer and disclosure of each individual's Protected Health Information (PHI).* The clinical notes signed by your doctor can be used in any court as a valid legal document, although hopefully that will never happen to you or any of your loved ones. These documents are kept for years either in a paper or paperless form. When you sign with a life insurance or health insurance and write your primary care doctor's name, the company will request copies of all your medical records which they use to place you in their pre-determined risk pools.

As a reminder, many health insurance companies still include a clause in the contract that denies coverage for pre-existing medical conditions. That is why they request your previous records from your primary care provider.

Another request for medical records that I've received many times comes from the Social Security Administration when someone applies for disability. The SSA uses the medical records as one of the criteria to establish the need for assistance.

In short, your medical record should be maintained in accordance with the law. You should have access to your record, and for a reasonable fee you can obtain a copy.

Before we depart from the medical records department let me clarify how most primary care physicians write their clinical notes on your chart.

SOAP

The part in the chart that documents your visit with the doctor is the clinical notes. Almost all clinical notes written by a primary care physician follow a universal four parts format that has been used and taught for years: "SOAP" (how can you forget that?) It's short for *Subjective* (the history you or others provide about your condition) *Objective* (the physical exam your doctor performs during the visit) *Assessment* (final diagnosis or impression) and *Plan* (the care plan for your diagnosis.) You already read about the first part, which is the medical history. If you think about the documentation you will find that it follows a problem solving logic. The first part (the history) is the problem that you are presenting to the doctor. The data included in the first part is entirely your version of the problem as you perceive it, so no matter how objective you are, to your doctor it is subjective. The second part of the encounter is objective to the doctor since she is conducting that task herself, see with her eyes, touch with her hands, and listen with her ears. It does not get any more objective than that.

The third part of the encounter documentation is the assessment or the problem name, in the problem solving model your doctor use subjective and objective data to find a diagnosis or name the problem. Once the problem is discovered then comes the final phase, the solution or in SOAP talks "the plan".

I will talk about the last three components more as we go along.

Back Desk and your satisfaction

You know if there's a front desk, there's got to be a back desk.

It took a while to understand the concept, partly because the name is artificial—it really labels functions more than an actual desk location. The front desk is for reception, while administrative duties and back desk are medical and clinical duties. I assume that medical staff offices got the name because they work in the back of the office.

You will notice that if you are asked to meet with your doctor or have a procedure done, you are moved to the back. This serves most people well because it allows for privacy.

The workers who staff the back desk may have a different medical education, experience and personality. Their role is to provide the doctor with technical (clinical) support by getting your vitals (temperature, weight, blood pressure) and writing down some elements of the clinical encounter, such as your chief complaints and concerns. They also will carry on with some of the doctor's plan of action, such as giving the shots or medication you need, obtaining a blood sample, performing a hearing or vision screen, hooking you up for an EKG, and so on.

Because their functions are very critical to your health, it is imperative you pay attention to their performance: did she get your blood pressure right? Did she hook the EKG machine up the proper way? Did she wipe your skin with alcohol before giving the shot? Each of these functions are being delegated to her by the doctor who trusts that all procedures are being performed not only to his satisfaction, but to your satisfaction as well.

I felt really bad one day when I had to fire a highly qualified and competent medical assistant. Although she did the procedures well, I received recurring complaints about her attitude, with one mother saying she was rude and another that she was condescending. I tried to work with her, but her personality was hard to change. Working hours and hours with demanding or distressed patients can be quite taxing on emotions and attitudes. Most medical staff develop survival coping techniques as they get into the field. But because you have the right to a professional, competent and courteous medical assistant, it is the office's responsibility to find her for you, then listen to your feedback and your perceptions of the service she provided.

At the end, remember that a competent and trained medical assistant should serve you during the visit by providing and performing procedures with respect and an attitude you find acceptable.

Examination Room and balloons

Hopefully you have found a way to avoid boredom during the time before the medical assistant or nurse calls your name and escorts you to the exam room. She will probably take your measurements, not like a tailor, but rather your weight, height, temperatures, blood pressure and heart rate. After recording all these vital signs in your chart, she will seat you in the exam room and ask you about your reason to see the doctor. After she concludes her task, she will leave you alone in the room, walking away and closing the door for your privacy. To many of my patients, this is the time when the fun begins, as the kids turn on the faucet, play with the soap dispenser, grab the paper towels, pull the napkin box or just climb up the walls. The expert child knows how to pull a glove or two from the glove box on the counter. When I enter the room I see happy child playing with balloon gloves, (If you're an adult, please don't do these acts; they are reserved for children.)

The walls in most new construction are thin enough for the staff to figure out what is happening behind closed doors. Spouses forget that sometimes and continue on with a quarrel from home which can be overheard. The clinic staff will protect your privacy as much as it is in their hands to do so, but if you decide to publicize your family arguments, there's not much they can do to help. One more thing: the stuff you see on the counter in covered glass containers should be left untouched both for your benefit and the benefit of other patients.

While waiting in the exam room, think of the encounter with your doctor as we eluded to it before as being in four parts. You've already prepared your S (subjective), the history part; the doctor will listen to what you have to say and proceed to the second part O (objective), or the physical exam.

Body Language

Before we get to the important topic of the physical exam, I would like to touch on the topic of body language. Some will refer to body language as non-verbal (non-written) communication. I can tell you that if a genius computer software designer ever invents a program to correctly interpret human body language, she will join the "Bill Gates" country club. Imagine a program that could tell the user what each look or gesture of the patient means, whether the patient is from Asia or Africa, male or female. Not like doctors who have to guess from heart rate and blood pressure, but something that actually translates non-verbal, non-written communication.

Why is body language so important in a doctor's office?

Simple, one of the biggest barriers to high-quality health care for millions of U.S. residents has nothing to do with medicine. It has to do with language. That is proven by research that states that between 1990 and 2000, the number of Americans speaking a language other than English at home grew by 15.1 million (a 47 percent increase) and the number with limited English proficiency grew by 7.3 million (a 53 percent increase). In other words we are looking at 50 million people in the U.S., 19 percent of the population, who speak a language other than English at home and 22 million who have limited English proficiency.

Research further showed that patients who face language barriers have difficulty accessing care, receive fewer preventive services, and are less likely to follow medication directions. For example, asthmatic children with language barriers are more likely to end up intubated in intensive care.

Non-verbal communication is the unofficial primitive messages we send to others all the time. If you have seen the 2005 Will Smith movie *Hitch*, you will know what I mean. Facial expressions, eye contact, hands and head movements, distance kept—all of these play a vital role during the physical examination and probably through your entire visit. As primary care physician offices attract more of a crowd than most specialty offices, there is frequent human interaction between different backgrounds. Non-verbal communications can be interpreted in many ways. The clinical encounter between you and your doctor is one between two humans, each of them observing the other.

The results of a study by Hall and Stein from the Department of Psychology at Northeastern University in Boston were puzzling. The study set out to assess primary care physicians' awareness of their patients' rated emotions, satisfaction, and opinion of the quality of their communication. The results showed a *substantial discrepancy* between physicians' and patients' opinion of how the doctor's visit went, such that physicians thought patients' responses were more negative than they actually were.

The key is that non-verbal communication can either corroborate your verbal communication or contradict it. It works in both sickness and in health. A 4-year-old child's grandmother gave me all the body language I needed to diagnose urinary tract infection in the young girl as I watched her imitation of the child's squeezing walk, holding her private parts and running to the bathroom. It was an imitation so good that it took less time for the encounter to conclude. On the other hand, I had a 16-year-old with all the body language of major depression, but her mom was in full denial, claiming "she's just here for her regular check up." But when I asked a couple more question, I received a different impression: the girl had lost all interest in talking to her friends on the phone, was having problem with sleep, hated leaving her room, thought she was ugly and even wanted to kill herself. Hello, I can see that depression when I walked into the room.

I learned from experience that watching the body language during the encounter is helpful to the examiner. I try to pay attention to the face and hands. Eye contact usually helps me determine how much of what I am saying is being absorbed, what I should repeat, and when should I stop. Many times it tells me if I am being accepted and allowed into the trust zone, or whether the head nodding is just a way to get the interaction over with quickly. As simple as this may sound, I tend to use the facial expressions of my patients or their parents to decide whether to say more, repeat what I said or stop all together.

You the patient or parent have the ability to fine-tune your interaction with your doctor. If you want to use your body language to explain your symptoms or complaints, go right ahead; some of my patients point to their right or left ear and moan or frown as soon as I enter the room to tell me "my ear hurts—do something."

Body language during the physical exam is even more important. I tell my patients all the time to tell me when my touch hurts, and almost always I can see that pain before I hear the *Ahh*. Even the quality of the pain (mild, moderate or severe) will be better reflected in the facial or body expression than in the *Ahh*.

I can also tell when my stethoscope is cold when my patients move away while I am trying to listen to the chest or heart. Working with children is a lot of fun when it comes to body language, as they are so transparent, easy to understand and straightforward with you.

To assure the reader that is not all about me and my experience, I would like to share what I found written in one of the professional magazines I read on regular basis. The article was titled "Handy tips can help speed things up in pediatric visits" it appeared in "Pediatric News" magazine vol. 40, No, 8 in August 2006.

The director of a busy children's hospital emergency room wrote that *watching a patient's eyes during physical examination can reveal a great deal.* He cited research done years ago that noted that among patients found to have *appendicitis* only 4% closed their eyes on physical exam, compared with 33% who did not have *appendicitis*.

The renowned professor of pediatrics also suggests asking the patient with suspected appendicitis to do a *"High five"* as those who refuse should be at risk of the disease.

Another expert pediatrician in the same article reminded us physicians that "Kids won't look up when their retropharyngeal space is filled with pus" which is a sign of bad infection in the patient's throat, yet sometimes can be easily missed by a physician.

Body language is also a tool for you to judge the confidence and the attitude of your doctor. Watching her body language, facial expressions and eye contact or recognizing if she has sweaty palms are all non-verbal clues to how the interaction is affecting her.

Now let me introduce you to the topic of physical exam:

<u>PHYSICAL</u>

In the primary care physician dictionary "Physical" is short for physical examination, It means just that. This is the part of the encounter where you are going to be looked at, touched and listened to. In medical textbooks it is Inspection, Palpation, Percussion and Auscultation. In many people's (especially adolescents') minds, it is the ultimate invasion of privacy. Read part 2, chapter one of Tolstoy's classic *Anna Karenina* and you will see what I mean.

The inspection means scanning the patient with the eyes only, it does give a chance to get a first impression; it is also a good warm up time for both of us before touching.

The palpation and percussion part of the exam involve light and deep touching, our hands and finger tips are equipped with dense nerve supply that help in defining things like rashes, masses, lumps, and of figure out where it hurts the most.

But I got to tell you the doctor's trade mark is auscultation "the famous stethoscope". People who know nothing but what they should know, and believe nothing but what they should believe perceive any human with a stethoscope as a doctor.

Many times during physical exam I find myself closing my eyes while performing the palpation or the auscultation part of the exam, I feel that I focus more on the body part I am examining.

The physical exam part of the encounter with your doctor is the next most important process to come to a conclusion. After listening to your version of the history, your doctor uses all her faculties for the objective part of the interview.

She will inspect with her eyes(sight and vision), touch with her fingers(tactile sensation), listen with her stethoscope(audio effect), and smell with her nose(sniff you illness).

One of my clinical instructors once told me years ago that he could diagnose streptococcal pharyngitis (strep throat infection) by just smelling the patient's open mouth. Now we prefer to use a test called strep screen to confirm such a diagnosis. Another cardiologist said he could diagnose those with sub acute bacterial endocarditis (a rare but serious heart infection) when he walked into the cardiac ward, as they have a different smell.

Having said all that, I bet you are going to take a shower before visiting your doctor, which is a great idea. The examination rooms now are small (economic) and closed, so although some have good ventilation, trust me you will notice when she enters the room whether your doctor forget her deodorant.

My Favorite Toys

In addition to using our own human senses, we like to utilize some fabulous toys, or at least that is what I tell the kids in my clinic. Those toys are tools just like the handyman uses as a doctor also needs a good flashlight, magnifying lens, measuring tape, and yes, sometimes a hammer. But of course, the trademark of a doctor is the famous stethoscope. I tell the children in my clinic I love to play with my toys, so that is what I do all day. You should see their reaction: some want so much to see what my other toys do that they don't want to go home. Just as the handyman carries his tools in a tool belt, I keep them in my white coat. The white coat is a protective outfit, tool belt and professional attire all in one. My toys are a little more expensive than others toys, but they are durable and reliable.

The conduct of the physical examination is sometimes methodical, starting from the top down, and sometimes focused, starting from the area of concern. Every practitioner develop his or her own protocol when it comes to physical examination. In my case as a pediatrician when I examine a toddler, I take the path of least resistance, I listen to the chest and heart, then inspect and feel the head and neck, I leave the ears until the end when the toddler doesn't have to be quiet and still. As looking at young kids' ears is associated eight times out of ten with anxiety, screaming and resistance may block any further advances by the examiner.

Professional resentment

What you will go through during a physical exam may involve all of your body organs and systems if your visit is for an annual check up, or just some of these organs if you're having a sick visit. I've previously mentioned the four steps we were taught in medical school (inspection, palpation, percussion and auscultation.) But there has been significant debate in the medical community for the past 15-20 years on the subject of physical exams. The old guard and the medical academia feel that physicians in the United States have been relying more heavily on the available, accessible technology to diagnose illnesses rather than the good old history and physical. Yet the teaching has never changed, as physicians still must use their clinical skills (collecting a good history and performing a proper physical exam) to diagnose illness. The use of investigations whether by blood sample, x-ray or MRI should be used only if necessary.

Along with the introduction of highly sophisticated blood analysis equipment and marvelous diagnostic radiology gadgets came the temptation to use and overuse the technology. Other factors are to blame, including defensive medicine, pressure to see more customers to make money, and the customer's (patient) pressure. When a mom came to my office with her child who had had symptoms of headache and dizziness for a couple of weeks, I did what I was trained to do by listening, examining, and reasoning as I tried to persuade her to accept my diagnosis of migraine. When she asked if we could get a

CT of his head, I explained that it was not only unnecessary, but might needlessly expose him to radiation. In short, I tried to detail the risk-versus-benefit model. She was convinced at the beginning, or at least I felt so. However, four week later I received a letter from a neurologist reporting that he had seen the child and diagnosed him with migraine after the MRI of the brain was negative. He concluded the child needed no medication other than what I had recommended in the first place. Two weeks later, the mother called me and.said she went to another neurologist at an academic institution who basically reached the same conclusion I had weeks ago. I use this example to give an idea of the kinds of pressure that primary care physician have to deal with on a daily basis.

The first disease that comes to a parent's mind when a school-age child complains of a headache is brain tumor. The first thing they would love for me to do is to get a head CT, although the odds of a brain tumor in a child are close to one in ten thousand. The incidence of tension headache or migraine in children is a hundred times more than a brain tumor. As the amount of radiation exposure during a head CT is much more than what you are exposed to during chest X-ray; there will always be potential risk from that exposure. It is even more serious if you need to undergo more CTs because the radiation accumulates. If this were my child, I would not choose to expose him to this risk at this stage.

Trust

The core issue is how much are you willing to trust your primary care physician? After doing a good job preparing for your visit, researching and making your selection, you need to trust in your own choice. If for whatever reason you don't trust your primary care physician, it will be unlikely that you will get the most benefit out of visiting her. I will never disagree with someone who wants to get a second opinion, but if that person ends up getting a second opinion time after time, I know there has to be something wrong in the relationship.

One of the sensitive and thorny issues that causes lots of confusion, debate, and suspicion is the issue of how long it takes a physician to perform a physical exam. The two most important factors are the patient's complaint (type of visit) and the physician's experience. As conscientiously as one can study during medical school and clinical residency, one still needs the daily practice experience to be efficient in the art of diagnosis.

My rash story

Let me tell you about the rash story. When I first started practicing after graduation, I was very good with serious, life-threatening, and rare illnesses. If the disease would lead to hospitalization, I knew every thing about it, from asthma, cystic fibrosis, and tumors to all the rest of horrible disease. But if it were some disease that needed only outpatient care, I hadn't spent enough time observing it, not to mention it usually was not as glamorous or flashy to dwell on during residency training. Even the pediatric board exam doesn't allocate high scores for the simple, common outpatient diseases the pediatrician encounters daily in practice.

Skin rash differential diagnosis was my weakness after graduation, as I spent a lot of time with each patient that showed up with a skin rash. However, I was lucky enough to work closely with a great dermatologist who used to come to our big clinic in Flint, Michigan and see all our patients who presented with skin problems (mostly rashes.) After spending hours with him, it took me much less time to diagnose and treat a skin rash.

The morale here is that experience has a significant impact on the time it will take for the physical exam.

Few months ago I attended a clinical conference in which a high profile renowned ophthalmologist "eye doctor" was teaching primary care physicians about eye examination and eye problems. He dared us to time him while he is performing a comprehensive primary care eye examination, it took him 90 seconds. He performed in those 90 seconds what a medical resident perform in about 900 seconds. I can see the glowing victory smile on his face when he proved his point to the audience.

In addition to experience, if during the annual check up your doctor happens to identify something unusual such as a heart murmur, cyst, or mole on your back, this incidental finding requires more time to scrutinize.

The mall and tools of the trade

Examination of certain body parts or organs requires specific instruments. To see your throat, I will need a good flashlight; to see your eardrums, I use an otoscope; to listen to your heart, I use a stethoscope. These tools of my trade are stored in my office since I am not in the habit of carrying them around every where I go.

One of my patient's mothers met me in a mall and asked if I could take a look at her son's throat to see if it was infected. I tried, but without a good flashlight, it just doesn't work. Therefore if you happen to run into your primary care physician in a mall, resist the temptation to ask for a free examination—it isn't worth it.

It is a two way street

You should realize the physical exam is an interactive process in which you should really give some sort of a feedback. When you are asked if something hurts, you ought to tell not only with a grimace, but speak up and be as specific as you can, saying whether it hurts that much, just a little, or really badly.

The same is true of the physician. When I first started my clinical rounds in medical school, my dad brought his sphygmomanometer home and asked me to examine his blood pressure. As I was busy wrapping the cuff around his arm and placing the stethoscope in my ears and anxiously listening to sounds of his heart pulsating, he suddenly noted, "you're not talking to me." I was surprised, but he said when you examine your patients, you have to talk to them. That was my first lesson of active interaction during physical examinations. Now I stress communication every step of the way during the patient visit because it's the secret to a good outcome. Verbal and non-verbal communication will get you the most out of your visit by making your complaints and concerns better understood by your doctor who can then provide you with more focused and guided instructions.

Normal or Abnormal: That is the Question

The strenuous training that medical students and residents have to undergo before graduation is intended in part to help with the task of separating normal findings from abnormal ones. Before I attended medical school, differentiating normal from abnormal was easy for me. My ears are normal, other people ears are not, my hands are normal and other people's hands are not. And without a doubt, the way I think is normal and you know others are just strange.

But when I first listened to heartbeats in my medical school class, I asked myself how in the world anyone could distinguish a first sound from a second sound, let alone try to figure out other normal and abnormal sounds. Yet our cardiology professor was quite confident that it was an easy task, as all you have to do is to listen to enough heart sounds and you will get the hang of it. He was right, although it did take years of practice, training and hundreds of hearts to get me to where I am (almost) confident to say this is a normal sound, an innocent murmur or one you better go see a cardiologist for evaluation. Most of us underestimate the value of knowing what is normal and what is abnormal whether in physical findings or emotions and feelings.

Normal variation is a concept I stress to many. One mom was very concerned and fretting over the surface appearance of her 2-year-old boy's tongue. She kept looking on the Internet for diseases and found that Systemic Lupus Erythematosus may cause tongue problems. The child was so normal I dared not expose him to the torture of blood samples or refer him to someone else who might. It took me a while, but her trust in me paid off; now two years later when she brings him for a physical, I tease her about how good his tongue looks right now, and she smiles and blushes.

Take height for example: short stature is a label for an abnormal condition, but it isn't one. As one of every 20 children is below the 5th percentile channel on a standard growth curve; in reality this is a statistical variation. Very few of those children who are falling below the standard height curve are truly abnormal and therefore need evaluation and treatment. However, from the statistical point of view, the number of abnormal stature cases among those who fall below the 5th percentile is relatively more when compared to those who fall between the 5th and 95th percentile channels. The same applies if you use the boundaries of 3rd and 97th percentile channels. Bedwetting is another issue I explain to parents is NORMAL for many children who wet the bed at night at age six.

What does that mean to you? If you hear from your doctor about an abnormal finding, whether physical or psychological, your next question is: how serious is it? Many parents panic when I say your child has an innocent murmur coming from the heart. Even though innocent should be self-explanatory, it takes a little bit of assurance to go over that concept. Many times the abnormal finding is actually normal for a particular person, as I explained earlier about height issues. But sometimes the abnormal finding is a warning or a marker for a more serious problem. A hearing loss can be the result of a transient and self-limited condition, meaning you get your full hearing back after the ear infection is gone, or a serious condition that threatens your health. I guess that part is taking us to the third component of the clinical encounter: the assessment or DIAGNOSIS

Diagnosis and related topics

The definition is simple: diagnosis is the art or act of identifying a disease from its signs and symptoms. As a reminder, here symptoms are reflected in the part we labeled as history or subjective, while signs are in the part we called objective, or the physical findings by your examining doctor. The diagnosis is the third part of the medical encounter's documentation. I think of this part as the climax of the encounter or the peak, as all the steps before it lead to it, while every step that comes after it descends from that peak. The care plan that follows a diagnosis of ear infection is much different from the care plan of an asthma diagnosis.

Your good doctor will use his knowledge, experience and assimilation of all the data he has learned from you and from his examination to reach that point. The achievement is to reach a correct diagnosis, one that ties up and explains all your problems that you presented to him earlier. Many times that process is a straightforward one; other times it becomes a challenge even for the best of doctors.

Barriers to clear cut diagnosis

The importance of a correct diagnosis is quite obvious, as every action and advice your doctor will offer to you depends on it being right. Yet if you ever get a chance to review clinical encounters written by physicians, you will find out how hard it can be to be sure.

1- Sometimes we use your symptoms as an inconclusive waste basket, e.g. cough, fever of unknown etiology, rash, headache and so on, as all these are really not what my old medical school professor would call a final DIAGNOSIS. As I was taught for years, a cough is a symptom, not a diagnosis. On the other hand, asthma is a diagnosis, so if I am positive that you are coughing because you're having an asthma attack, then I have a diagnosis. If I say cough, that entails that at this point I will ask for other tools to help me make the diagnosis later on. But for the purpose of complying with the standard format of SOAP, I have to fill in the "A" or the diagnosis part.

2- More than one diagnosis may be needed to explain your complaints. My old medical school professors hated that, because the old way of teaching was that if you could tie all the symptoms up in one bundle and label it with one disease, you were a good doctor. As I have been practicing for years, I am no longer convinced of that philosophy any more, as in my mind it is an oversimplification of the process rather than finding the truth. I admit that throughout the history of medicine, dedicated, smart physicians have discovered many diseases such as cystic fibrosis, systemic Lupus, Marfan syndrome, and others by following and caring for patients closely. But statistically speaking, the odds of having a child with a cough and diarrhea is much likely to be due to two different common viruses (RSV and Rotavirus) i.e. two diseases, than cystic fibrosis i.e. one disease.

3- The stages. Many people have hard time understanding the concept of DISEASE STAGES. For so many diseases, whether acute like flu or chronic like asthma and diabetes, there are always stages. The dilemma here is that each stage may present itself in a different and sometimes deceiving manner, while each stage needs targeted treatment. Asthma is a great example of the camouflage that certain diseases put on, as most people with mild asthma cough or wheeze only once in a while. If different doctors see them each time, it will be hard for a particular one to pick up on the pattern and make the correct diagnosis. In my experience (and I am sure in the experience of others), I've seen patients who have lived for years with asthma but never gotten the diagnosis at the right time.

You want to learn about another problem, let me take you to DIFFRENTIAL DIAGNOSIS.

Differential Diagnosis

Imagine yourself at the movies where 100 actors are playing the same role, saying the same lines. Can you identify and name each actor?

But that's how overwhelmed a medical student feels when a clinical instructor asks a question of differential diagnosis. I typed the term *skin rash* on my Internet search engine; it came up with 11,300,000 web sites. When I typed *cough*, it gave me "only" 3,400,000 web sites. There are extensive lists of diseases for each complaint, symptom, and medical problem you can ever imagine. Some are organized and some are not. Doctors in training spend hours and hours learning about differential diagnosis every day, in morning rounds, noon conferences, grand rounds and board review classes.

Differential diagnosis is also one of the cores of medical education. That's the reason I'm surprised at people trying to treat their symptoms without seeing a doctor by just going to the pharmacy or reading a book. I had a parent in my clinic that spent $35 on cough medicines, but after I examined his son, I told him to throw all of them in the trash as none was appropriate for his child's condition.

To make even more fun, some less common conditions may masquerade as very common ones. Right at the peak of the stomach flu (viral gastroenteritis) season, I had a 7-year-old boy coming in with vomiting, diarrhea and some abdominal discomfort. That is a straightforward diagnosis I thought, as I had diagnosed many children over the last few weeks with this and they did great. But while I was examining him, I noticed he was in more pain than usual for his age with this condition, so I kept him a little longer. As I examined his two other siblings in the room with him, I kept telling myself he was sicker than normal. After I sent him to the ER, I got a call few hours later that he was proven to have appendicitis and was taken to the OR for surgery that night. Mind you if you look in the medical textbook, it will mention that constipation rather than diarrhea is one of the presenting symptoms for "appendicitis." So how do you like differential diagnosis now?

The Misdiagnosis Trap

I wish I could tell you that you don't have to worry about the nasty term *misdiagnosis*, but you are probably smarter than that. To err is human—to misdiagnose you have to practice medicine. Doctors who never practice regular patient care will never misdiagnose any disease. Yet a plaintiff's medical expert witness in a malpractice lawsuit will try to persuade the jury that misdiagnosis is an unforgivable crime.

Every good doctor and every health care consumer including you should worry about misdiagnosis. I was in a lecture last night where the research psychiatrist told us a sad story about a

17-year-old who had been treated for years for Attention Deficit and Hyperactivity Disorder, after thorough re-evaluation by the research psychiatrist (he was being held in detention), he was found to have classic schizophrenia. Every doctor stores in his memory bank many stories of misdiagnosis. One of the patients that came to me with a diagnosis of moderate asthma was proven to have a genetic condition called Cystic Fibrosis. I have treated many children who scratched their skin for month and were treated for eczema, but they actually had an infection with scabies. A long time ago I worked with a pediatrician who lost a malpractice case for misdiagnosing a foreign body in a child's airway. He was treating the child for asthma.

Misdiagnosis is a fact of life where doctors should take their share of the blame, but we need informed consumers who are willing to change the system. I wish someone could actually put a dollar figure on the cost of misdiagnosis in our health care. If you ask for a wild guess, it must be billions of dollars per year. Misdiagnosis should not be confused with differential diagnosis; the latter is a laundry list of conditions that must be sorted out for the physician to reach the correct diagnosis. Working with a differential diagnosis is good practice, but working with a misdiagnosis is bad. My guiding principle to avoid misdiagnosis is simple. I expect my patient to respond favorably to the treatment as expected, or else we both have to work harder to find the truth.

There is another term you need to learn about to get better information from your doctor's visit: *ETIOLOGY.*

MAHMOUD ELGHOROURY, MD, FAAP

Etiology and Tricks of the trade

Etiology in short is all of the causes of a disease or abnormal condition. This is not the same as diagnosis, so it can get confusing. To make it clear, let's say your diagnosis is asthma; the etiology here is a combination of a genetic predisposition and your immune response to other factors. For a diagnosis of ear infection, the etiology can be a viral or bacterial organism. The same can be said for sinus or throat infections. The wide world of etiology is more fascinating and intriguing than the World Wide Web as it takes from everything from the universe of microorganisms to the mystery of immune systems. You travel through the history of genetics, chromosomes and DNA, or the maze of hormones and their complex control systems.

The term will come up when you ask your doctor after his evaluation and diagnosis: how (why) did that happen to me?

Most people expect a straightforward and easy answer to that simple question, but the vast current knowledge base in medicine and science may challenge that expectation.

In medical school teachings and medical textbooks we organize the etiology of a disease or a disorder (diagnosis) into categories such as:

1- Infections: bacterial, viral or parasitic.
2- Immune or autoimmune dysfunction.
3- Inherited or genetic disorder.
4- External factors such as toxins, smoking, injury (recent or old.)
5- Nutritional, excess of one nutrient (excess fat), or lack of another (Vitamin deficiency.)

6- Hormone (endocrine) related, such as diabetes or thyroid problems.

7- Tumors, benign or malignant.

8- Psychological or mental, such as depression.

9- Other, undetermined, or unknown. (I'm sure you hate that as much as I do, as it is a humbling block.)

10- Iatrogenic, the malpractice lawyer's favorite. I don't need to say anymore of what that means do I? The etiology of the illness is due to doctor's error.

11- Combination of two or more of the above etiologies.

Many times it becomes difficult to pinpoint the exact cause of one's problem, complaint or symptoms (diagnosis.) For example, we know that many organisms are capable of producing ear infection, but which one of the many infective organisms is it in a particular case? For the available technology to identify a specific organism is very limited compared to the colossal number of known infective ones. But we may be able to use research or advanced technology to identify the organism in special circumstances.

Even if one is diagnosed with a very specific virus such as flu or infectious mononucleosis, does the etiologic diagnosis explain all the symptoms?

I have seen many adolescents who presented with symptoms indicative of infectious mononucleosis (caused by the Epstein-Barr virus) who tested positive for the disease. Many followed the expected natural course of the disease and had no problem, recovering within days and going back to school and their daily routine. On the other hand, a few had a troubling course from persistent fever to a spreading rash or lack of energy and weight loss that dragged on for weeks. The offending agent was exactly the same.

A tricky one occurs when someone presents with a sore throat and his strep test is positive; as most will conclude that the streptococcal (bacterial) infection is the etiology of the sore throat; therefore once treated with antibiotics, it will be resolved. But current medical knowledge proves that simple and logical assessment is not always true, as in some cases, the person has been carrying the strep bacteria all along(without being sick) and it just happened that when she got a viral infection that actually caused the swollen red throat and the illness, she went to the doctor and complained. The physician then order the strep test, and with positive strep test and clinical symptoms he is sure that etiology of the patient's disease is the strep bacteria. The true etiology is a viral infection of the throat and the strep bacteria just happened to be there.

For the most part though, with our ever-expanding medical knowledge, we think the etiology of many diseases can be identified and explained to the patient. That is why you still have to ask the question: what is the cause of my problems? Or why did this happen to me? If you know, in the future you may be able to take precautions to save yourself from having to come back to the doctor.

Tied to diagnosis and etiology is the subject of PROGNOSIS.

Prognosis and Weather predictions

What is prognosis? Well, prognosis is the prospect of recovery as anticipated from the usual course of the disease. We talk about it in terms of GOOD, BAD, UGLY or in-between. Actually I'm just kidding, as real doctors' use only professional words such as *good*, *fair*, *poor*, or *unknown* prognosis (here is the hated unknown again.)

This is what you would call an educated guess. Based on professional experience and knowledge, it predicts for the patient the most likely outcome and course of a specific condition. Your viral illness is predicted to have a good prognosis as you are likely to feel better in 3-5 days. In other words do not worry much and take it easy, which sounds good to all. Say, have you ever compared the weather predictions you see on the news a week ahead to the real weather when it hits? A doctor's prognosis is close enough, but while meteorologists use radars and satellites, we use stethoscopes and hammers. They analyze their database while we look at textbooks.

For a prognosis to be valid, certain things must be assumed:

1- The diagnosis is correct.
2- There are no other unknown or underlying problems that may alter the prognosis, e.g. getting another infection on top of the first one or having a weak immune system.
3- The instruction for treatment is followed, including proper rest, proper fluid and fever management.

You have to pay attention to the prognosis part of the visit, so ask questions if you're not sure. As this is a crucial part of the clinical encounter between the patient and the doctor, there should be no misunderstanding. Also as I explain to my patients, if the prognosis I'm telling you doesn't materialize I need to know about it.

Many parents bring their children in after they've had a runny nose and fever for a couple of days. After I'm sure of the diagnosis of simple viral upper respiratory infection, as I summarize I will say that your child should feel better within 5-7 days; therefore IF her symptoms persist or get worse, please let me know. Many times a mild upper respiratory infection may lead later to bacterial middle ear infection or sinus infection where antibiotics will be needed for treatment

Plan of Care or Solution

Now that we talked about S, O, and A, S for (subjective or history), O for (objective or physical exam) and A for (assessment or diagnosis, it's time to take you to the next part of the clinical encounter, the "P" plan of care, which is tailored for you. As I mentioned earlier another way to think of the clinical encounter is to compare to a problem solving exercise. In the problem solving model the plan of care is *"The Solution"*. The plan of care includes every action done after the diagnosis, including taking a blood sample, ordering an X-ray, asking for a second opinion, etc.

After listening to you, examining you, and diagnosing you as having or not having an illness, your physician has to formulate a plan specific for you and your condition. If you are in a perfect health, you get a pat on the back and told to keep doing what you are doing....*but*. The *but* is the plan, as she will tell you things like twenty minutes of walking each day is good for you, or you may want to get out of the office more often. Many times you need to modify some of your eating habits or learn about a new risk factor that may threaten your health now or in the future.

Your doctor may discuss with you the need for a blood test, X-ray, or referral to a specialist. The part of the plan that most of us don't use is the counseling part.

By now your doctor knows specific medical details about you—information just you and she share. Rather than asking questions in general about obesity or blood pressure or asthma, ask a question about how a condition or problem affects YOU. What does she think you should do about your problem? The Internet is filled with all kinds of information about any disease you will ever imagine, so you can always go back and look up the disease that you're interested in, but here in the office, face to face with YOUR physician, ask how that condition or this disease will affect YOU. What should you do to get better? What is the best medicine for you?

For each condition or disorder in general there are different severity scales, as different factors may influence that particular disease progression or prognosis and outcome.

If you feel overwhelmed, it is better to listen and get the bottom line information, but do keep the line of communication open with your physician. Most of us will be happy to answer your written questions when you bring them to the following visit.

If you feel surprised about what your doctor said, ask for a second opinion. Use the knowledge of more than one doctor when you need to.

The plan is composed of the counseling you receive from your doctor regarding your diagnosis, including both the short- and long-term risks involved. It includes any specific investigation she may request (blood sample, X-ray, etc.) It also includes the medications she prescribes and procedures she wants you to go through before leaving the office (for example, having an EKG.) She will also use a phrase such as "call back with any problem or concern" or "report if the condition worsens."

The last component of the plan is the follow-up date. Does doctor have a scientific way to tell you exactly what day you should come back for a follow up on your condition? Sometimes we do, but most of the time, we do not. An annual check up is easy as it means making one visit per year from age 2 and up, but after that I've found no strict evidence for setting the follow-up appointment interval. Say you came in for diabetes: if you're doing a good job of managing it, you may come back in 3 - 6 months, but if your blood sugar level is not as good as it should be, you probably need to follow up sooner. If your child had a severe ear infection with loss of hearing, it makes sense that I should see him sooner than the other one who just had a mild infection. Many times I just leave the door open; if you're doing well and the problem is solved, just call me back or come in if you need to. This attitude is permissible if the treating physician gains enough confidence in her patient that the patient will follow the plan to the letter. For obvious reasons of medical legal liability, this option is left to each physician's judgment. Bottom line, if you trust your physician and she trusts you, you get to save time and money. Some of the future visits can also be avoided by a phone call. And by the way, I have never met a physician who got paid for a phone consultation, while a lawyer will charge for every minute on the phone.

Now let me give you some more insight on what I just summarized. We'll talk about some items that will show up on your care plan menu.

Let me introduce you to an important item on the menu of your care plan:

Testing – Investigation and the Sensitivity Factor

You doctor may perform certain tests in the office or refer you to outside health facilities. The following are simple rules for you to remember while in the office.

1- Simple tests and investigations that are done in most primary care physician's offices include things like routine blood tests, strep screen, EKG, X-ray, vision or hearing tests. In general, many of these tests will be billed to you or your insurance company over and above the charge for your sick or well visit. It is usually added to the doctor's visit charge

2- You should be informed of what tests your doctor is requesting and why they are needed.

3- In the event your insurance doesn't cover a test, ask the staff (front desk) what kind of financial options are available to you. Many offices will offer a discount for upfront cash payment (it does save the office the cost of paper or computer billing if you pay upfront.)

4-   What if you don't agree to the test? Remember it is ultimately your decision to consent to any test or procedure being suggested by your doctor. I like people who ask because it makes the job easier as the explanation allows for better interaction and understanding. I tell some parents and patients it forces you to buy into the program. When some asked why I want to do a strep test, I say if it is negative, it will spare you the antibiotics. Another example is if I don't know how high your blood cholesterol level may be, I won't be able to advise you of your risk of heart disease or the benefit of using medication to help lower your cholesterol.

5-   If you know that you've been tested for the same reason recently in a different office, tell that to your doctor as she may have overlooked some of your previous records.

6-   Refrain from being your own doctor. You have chosen a doctor that you trust, so don't manipulate her to order a certain test your friend suggested to you. Every now and then I get requests from parents asking for a head CT or MRI if the child complains of headache, or chest X-ray if the child is coughing. For each investigation or test, there must be a good reason to order it—i.e. a good chance it will yield helpful information that affects the management of your condition. More investigations, lab tests or X-rays do not guarantee better care. The cost and the risks of doing each particular test should be justifiable and reasonable as well as understood by you. Many times ordering a test that was not needed leads to a finding that is not relevant (meaningless.) Yet that irrelevant finding may require more testing, which ultimately costs a lot while still leading to nothing.

For years I cared for two sisters who were brought to my care after being diagnosed with a very rare disorder. The parents told me they had been taking their kids to doctors and hospitals since birth because of rashes, ear infections and cold symptoms. They had done EXTENSIVE testing and finally found an abnormal lab value. A renowned chief of a pediatric gastroenterology department in one of the most prestigious teaching institutions in the country made the diagnosis based on that one test (because all others were normal) along with the parents' description of their girls' history. To make a long story short, after multiple ER visits to many hospitals and admissions to every local hospital, I persuaded the ER physician to transfer the girls back to the renowned teaching institution (mind you I had received mountains of records and consultations regarding two girls who looked healthy every time I'd seen them in the office.) Ten days later one famous pediatrician from the same institute confirmed to me my worst fear when she labeled the situation as Munchhausen by Proxy, a condition in which the parents exaggerate or fake symptoms to seek medical care. But she could not proceed with the full management because of the label the Chief of Pediatric Gastroenterology had used to diagnose the children. The girls then were taken off the unneeded mineral supplement. The final outcome was the girls are in good shape with no meds, but the parents went through a bitter divorce. Lesson to you: don't ask for what you don't need, as you may get what you won't like.

The types of investigations your doctor will order differ in many ways. Investigations are divided in general into invasive and non-invasive categories.

1- Invasive would be like taking a biopsy from your kidney or your liver, or introducing a scope to your stomach. It means an invasion of your body one way or another. As you can tell, these tend to be a big deal and cost a bundle, so you really need to ask good questions about how much of a difference that procedure will make to your condition.

2- Non-invasive are in general less of a hazard, but they're not risk-free as even with the best technology, there is significant radiation exposure with CTs. If you are young, the exposure to radiation is cumulative, meaning the more frequently you or your child is exposed to radiation, the higher the risk of future illnesses, specifically malignant tumors, leukemia and others.

One thought to keep in mind is the concept of test sensitivity and specificity. The sensitive test should pick up the diseases diagnosis when performed, so the higher the test sensitivity the better the test. Specificity is almost the opposite; the test *should not* pick up the Diagnosis when it does not exist. In short a good test or investigation should have a high sensitivity score like 90% and a high specificity score to be reliable. Unfortunately many tests are not that good in the specificity and the sensitivity department.

Another hot item on your care plan may be a referral.

Referrals and Nightmares

You go to your primary care physician, who determines that your condition needs the expertise of a specialist, so she refers you to one. Well, at least that was the case in the good old days before the age of HMO dominance. Then I used to tell my assistant that this patient needs an ENT (Ear Nose and Throat) surgeon, so please give her the phone number for his office. The deal took no more than two minutes.

I still remember vividly the agonizing change I witnessed in Flint, Michigan while I was employed by a big multi-physician group. In the early 1990s, the HMO storm hit that practice full force. All of sudden most of the patients were enrolled in one HMO or another, and the word *referral* became a nightmare for our nurses, administrators, physicians and patients.

HMOs have a formal process for referrals that involves paperwork, faxed documents, network limitations, medical necessity determination and a review committee if needed. Angry phone calls from patients were being handled by frustrated staff who were struggling to understand and work with the change. Administrators had a hard time absorbing the needed cost for additional staffing just to handle referrals. Weekly and monthly staff meetings were basically dedicated to coming up with solutions for the avalanche of problems created by the change.

As by now the change has settled in, most offices accept the process as a routine one. The staff knows what forms to use, whom to call and so on. The HMO does retain the right to reject a referral if the medical condition is not meeting their criteria, which then starts the appeals process. However, unless you're planning to work in a doctor's office, you don't need to know about the headaches that come with appeals.

What you must know is your insurance policy for referral, including their network and restrictions. Each has its own manual and handbook that you will be delighted to know changes at least once year, and yes, NO TWO HMOs are exactly alike.

Medications and the Rules

Before you get bored, I will take you to an exciting item on your plan menu, one you have been waiting for all along: MEDICATION.

Medications are an integral part of health care, as throughout history people have believed in their healing power. Before surgical procedures were invented, it was all about medication. Potions, powders, creams, and ointment were all secrets wizards and magicians learned to use. And don't forget the poisons, some of which can heal as well as kill. It was all-natural then as there were no giant pharmaceutical corporations or Food and Drug Administration. No TV commercials and no sales representatives, so medications were kept in natural containers rather than colorful boxes with written instructions and warnings. In the good old days no one had committees and policies to prevent medication errors. But hey, enough of this old talk—let me bring you forward to our time.

There are general rules about today's medications that I would like to stress here:

1- As there has never been a risk-free medicine, you need to ask if the risk of taking a medicine is justified.

2- All medications have the potential to provoke an allergic reaction. Yes, some will do that even if you have taken them before and nothing happened. If you have ever reacted to any medication (hives or skin rash, stomach upset or vomiting, swelling, or even worse, had difficulty breathing), let the office staff know from the receptionist to the medical assistant. Let your pharmacist know too, as she will keep this information in her central computer for eternity.

3- Some medications have a special risk profile for certain people. If you have a sick kidney, liver failure, blood clotting problem, or any other chronic condition, make sure your doctor is aware of it.

4- If you are not sure about the instructions regarding how, when and for how long to take your medication, don't leave the office puzzled. Even if you used it in the past, ask until you know exactly how to use the medicine properly.

5- Try to use one pharmacy to fill all your prescriptions, as most pharmacies now employ sophisticated technology that can help prevent medication errors and avoid harmful interactions between different medications. The key is most of them are using their own data, so if you go to more than one pharmacy, you may not be able to get the benefit of these advanced software programs.

6- If you learn about a new medicine from commercial TV ads, it will be an expensive one, *guaranteed.*

7-   Over-the-counter (OTC) medications may sometimes
      interact with prescription drugs, so tell your prescriber
      what OTC medications or herbs you're using.

When you take the medicine from the pharmacist, review
the complete information label from your name to the drug
name and dosage. I've experienced a few instances where
either the pharmacist made a mistake or my handwriting was
confusing that resulted in either a wrong medicine being given
or a wrong dosage suggested. Thank God no harm was done,
but anxieties about medication errors are mounting for a good
reason, as they are a real and dangerous threat. The National
Coordinating Council for Medication Error Reporting and
Prevention (NCC MERP), an independent body comprised of
22 national organizations, defines a medication error as "any
preventable event that may cause or lead to inappropriate
medication use or patient harm while the medication is in the
control of the health care professional, patient, or consumer.
Such events may be related to professional practice, health
care products, procedures, and systems, including prescribing;
order communication; product labeling, packaging, and
nomenclature; compounding; dispensing; distribution;
administration; education; monitoring; and use."

For more information on the subject you can go to the
FDA web site, www.fda.gov

I would like to share with you an illustrative story I heard
from a well-seasoned pulmonologist (specialist in lung and
breathing problems) who practiced for decades. He told us
primary care physicians the story during a medical conference
about asthma management. The mother of a high-ranking
politician was referred to him after failing to respond to many

medications to treat her asthma. He reviewed her case and medications and wondered why she wasn't responding. He then took the time to watch her personally use her inhalers (asthma medications) and realized she was doing it wrong. Finally he told us that's the first thing he does whenever he hears a story like this, as one of the most common reasons of failing to respond to asthma medications is improper use.

You may think that taking a pill is easy, as it involves nothing more than throwing it in your mouth, swallowing, and washing it down with some water. But there are some medications that work only if taken on an empty stomach. I remind the patients who get tetracycline antibiotic pills to take them two hours before meals. Others must be after a meal, on a full stomach. Some you must chew; others you must place under your tongue.

The bottom line is medications are not going to work for you unless you both use them and use them right.

Before I depart from the medication department, I feel compelled to tell you about the PLACEBO EFFECT. The dictionary defines this as "improvement in the condition of a sick person that occurs in response to treatment but cannot be considered due to the specific treatment used." The term was coined and used extensively since 1950. I first experienced it while in middle school, as a worker in my grandfather's factory used to suffer occasional severe renal colic from a kidney stone. The pain always responded well to a medication that was prescribed to my grandmother for the same condition. One morning after seeing him in agonizing pain, I told my uncle, who a few minutes later gave him a small pill and told him it was my grandmother's wonder medicine. Ten minutes later the worker was back on his feet, grateful to my uncle and grandmother. But as I looked at my uncle while we were going back to the house, I saw this sly smile on his face. He told me that because he couldn't find my grandmother's prescription, he'd given the guy only a fake white pill that had no real medicine in it. It wasn't until I was introduced to the placebo effect in medical school that I figured out why the pain nonetheless disappeared. It's the power of the mind over body, almost like hypnosis.

This means all drugs must be tested and compared to the placebo effect before being submitted for FDA approval. The fact is that for almost every drug on which research has been done, from pain killers to antibiotics to skin creams, the placebo effect is so real as to be mind-boggling. Many people ask me about herbal supplements, vitamins and additive that allegedly do miracles. The advertisement will inform you that this non-prescription magical treatment for hair growth or fighting obesity works so well that you'll get your money back if it doesn't. In my opinion, those guys would never be in business if it wasn't for the amazing *placebo effect.* I invite you to think about that whenever you hear or see a commercial about seaweed or another ancient, recently rediscovered recipe. At least do yourself a favor and look at their research database to see if they controlled for the placebo effect. (If you are a fiction storywriter, try it as a title for your next best seller.)

I know I should leave the medication item, but one more thing more: BLACK BOX warnings. If you are not interested, skip this part, but you really should know something about the black box warning. NO, it is not the part they search for when a plane crashes—it's a written warning mandated by the FDA. In fact it is the strongest caution from the FDA to prescribers and patients regarding possible adverse effects of certain medication. When you see a black box warning, make sure you read it carefully, and if you have questions about it, talk to your doctor (not the receptionist.)

Shots and Fear

Now I need to take you to an item on the menu that everyone hates, including me: shots/ immunizations. I feel like I'm in a hot pressure cooker when I hear about attacks on children's immunization practices. I talk about my personal experience growing up in Egypt watching so many people paralyzed from the polio infection. My best friend's cousin lost the use of his left leg from that disease; as he grew older he worked out, and every muscle in his body bulged like a body builder except his atrophied leg. He refused to use a cane or crutch, just his hand to move his paralyzed leg. Although it was inspiring to see how he conquered his disability, I have seen the other tragic effects of infections from vaccine-preventable diseases. Something that is crippling and sometimes deadly to the children: what could be worse? Just try to meet with those children's parents, look in their eyes, and feel the agony. The devastating loss of one's child is an unbearable pain to parents who have to go on living and remembering.

As I worked as a resident in the emergency room, I've seen those who came in with dreadful signs of meningitis (brain infection.) On the hospital wards I cared for babies who suffered from pneumonia (lung infection) or couldn't breathe on their own. I wish we had a vaccine for every infection, for that will be the true advancement in medicine. In my opinion, the best difference between the medicine we practice now and medieval medicine is our ability to vaccinate and keep at least some of these devastating ailments from occurring.

Yet as I was trying to persuade one of the mothers to vaccinate her baby, she said she had been listening to different people who told her that the pediatricians' advice to vaccinate is *tainted* because they work in the field. I thought that was funny: if I advised her about fashion or make-up, would she then take my advice because it wouldn't be *tainted?*

As you can tell by now, I am a very strong advocate of vaccination. Having said that, I hate with passion the fearful looks of some of my patients when they see those needles. What I hate even more is that although I'm doing what I believe to be essential for their well-being, *I* invoked that fear directly or indirectly. Many grow up and forget or even they become my friends as time passes, but not all of them. You may need to receive a medication or immunization via an injection, which is painful either way. But the anticipation and the waiting is more annoying; ask me as I deal with it many times every day.

I dared to give my own four children their infant and toddler vaccinations, but it was not without a price. Sometimes I personally administered them, while sometimes my medical assistant would do it. I never had a problem until I needed to give my teenage daughter her booster shot. All of a sudden as I was injecting the immunization, she turned very pale, and a few seconds later she was on the floor of my clinic unconscious.

This is a condition that happens to many people during anxious events which is called a vaso-vagal attack. I've learned to ask both parents and older children if they're going to faint when they see or get the shots. If the answer is yes, I ask them to lie flat on the exam table or leave the room (if they don't need to be with the child) providing another guardian is available. If they're the ones getting the shot, I ask them to think pleasant thoughts or ask if they feel they would rather go home and come back when their mind is willing to handle the fear. Bleonophobia, fear of needles (or "needle phobia" as I call it) is more common than most people think. Some even scream when the area of skin where the needle will be injected is being numbed with an anesthetic patch!

Counseling

Counseling is the least utilized item on the menu of your care plan. You are now in a great hurry to grab the prescription and run out of the office so you can go on with your life. But did you happen to learn what the expert who examined you has to say about how YOU can help yourself stay healthy? Counseling is your underutilized opportunity to get specific answers about your own health from your doctor, face to face. Walk out of the office with some missing information and you will have to call back, wait on the phone or take a number.

The last entry most physicians write in the SOAP notes is the follow-up plan.

The term *follow-up* can be quite tricky for those lucky ones who only see their physician once a year for a physical. The doctor's obligation to you when she makes a diagnosis and formulates/designs a care plan for you, including medicine or a request for an X-ray, is to confirm that YOU responded to her management plan—that you are cured and back to normal. So if she says, "it looks like you just have a cold, but call me if you ***do not*** feel better in a week or if you are feeling ***worse***," that last part is her follow-up plan. Otherwise if you recover, as far as she's concerned your case is closed.

That is the part that creates much confusion to many. You may or may not be asked to come back at a specific time (day, week, or month) for a follow-up visit. But just because you're not asked to come back doesn't mean you shouldn't come back if in a few days you're still not feeling better. Just like with the weather, the dark clouds may stay around longer than predicted.

For certain symptoms such as headache and coughing, if they annoy you for a few days but then resolve themselves, that's one thing; but if you have the symptom for weeks, that's a different story. Follow-up visits in these cases are sometimes more important than the initial visit to lead your doctor to the correct diagnosis or care plan, especially for symptoms that are quite common such as cough, fever, headache, and so on.

Now that we are done with the SOAP, let me tell you about some perks that you may take advantage of when you are still in the office.

Visit Perks

Samples

One of the perks of having a personal physician who cares about you and is willing to go the extra mile to help is medication samples. A mother called me last night who had taken her son to the ER for swimmer's ear. Her insurance refused to cover the $75 prescription written by the ER staff physician. I told her that I had samples in my office and if she stopped by in the morning, I would give her some.

Prescription medications are either affordable or expensive. Almost all the new medications many of you have seen on TV commercials are expensive. The cost of buying these drugs can be really staggering whether you need to use them for a short period or for a long time to come. Even with traditional insurance that covers new medications, the co-pay for non-generics can be a burden. For example, one of my patients had a $40 co-pay for a 5-day course of eye drops.

The pharmaceutical companies use the doctors to market their products. After all, doctors are the ones who can make it happen, as they are the ones who will eventually push either drug A or drug B. One of the many marketing tools the companies use to persuade a doctor to prescribe a particular drug for patients (who may or may not be able to afford it) is to load up the office with free samples. Each office had a closet full of medication samples as pharmaceutical companies send their representative to keep them fully stocked. As in every business, you know the goal of this free program: get you (the consumer) to try it, like it and use it. But let me share with you the good news:

1- If you have insurance that will pay for a brand name drug but with a backbreaking co-pay, the drug representative may leave coupons in the office to absorb most or all of your co-pay.

2- If you have no insurance or your medical insurance doesn't cover that particular drug, the drug representative may deliver enough samples to the office to spare you some or even all of the cost of buying it all together.

3- If you qualify for one of the pharmaceutical assistance programs, the company may deliver the medicine to your place, sometimes free of charge. The details are usually left at your doctor's office.

On many occasions I have given away to my patients not only expensive brand prescription medications, but over-the-counter brand name cold, fever or pain medicines. As a pediatrician, I even get a lot of formula samples for new mothers who cannot breast- feed their babies. (As a note here, I do believe wholeheartedly that breast milk is the best for all babies unless strong reasons make it impossible.)

Vaccines for Free

Another perk that your child will benefit from in visiting her primary care physician is free vaccinations for children 18 years or younger. This federal program started in the mid-1990s is called Vaccine for Children (VFC); it's one of the best federally funded programs I've ever seen as it provides all vaccines necessary to protect children from birth to 18 years of age including the flu vaccine. Some of these vaccines render protection for years and some for even decades. I still get parents who call me in a panic when their child has a rash and fever as they're worrying about measles. Fortunately because of the prevalence of measles vaccines, I can calm them down instantly by saying, "the odds of your child having measles are one in a million." In 2003, the State of Michigan Health Department confirmed only two cases of measles in the whole state. One was a 9-month-old and the other was 25. This is remarkable considering the population of Michigan is close to 9 million.

Although the VFC program was started during a Democratic presidency, it has lasted for years now under a Republican one. This program has made a remarkable difference in the vaccination ratio among children, and in my mind has saved thousands of lives and billions of dollars. It protected millions from crippling diseases that have permanently damaged so many lives in the past from paralyzing polio to lethal brain infections.

Did it also help adults? You bet. Think about this for a minute: you go home when your child is sick with flu. As you live with her, care for her, and feed her, the odds are you're also going to get the flu. Apply the same rule to chicken pox, which is a relatively mild disease when young kids get it, but when adults are infected they get an extremely painful disease called shingles. If your child is immunized against chicken pox, the odds are less that you or other adults in the household will get the infection. Many surveys and studies have proven beyond any reasonable doubt that the benefits from immunizing children have also spread to adults.

CHAPTER FOUR
Exit

Finally you are walking out of the office, back in your clothes, with no hospital or medicinal smells surrounding you. As you pass the exit sign in a hurry to resume your regular daily chores and routines, you want to forget the whole encounter and the experience of being in the doctor's office. Hey, but remember the goal we started with—get the most of the doctor's visit—so you shouldn't stop here. There's just a few more steps to take. The relief you feel when an anticipated event like this is over shouldn't hold you back from the next step.

Before you retreat back into your comfort zone, ask the real question about how you feel regarding your doctor: if I cheated on my wife and thought I might have a sexually transmitted disease, could I confess that to my primary care physician? If the answer is *no*, you're in trouble; if the answer is only *maybe*, think harder. The correct answer has to be an unequivocal *yes*. Your own health and the health of others may one day depend on the correct answer.

There is a good primary care physician waiting for you, so go and find him. How do I know? Because I've worked with so many PCPs who honored their patients' trust, lived up to their expectations, and delivered the best professional care there is.

This is as real as California's sunshine every day. The good follow-up process starts here.

Follow-up Step One: Think.

Think, Replay

The first thought after you leave the office should be about the doctor. What is your feeling about her? Re-play the interaction part in your mind from different angles and zoom in and out with your mind's eye for a few minutes. Analyze your perception of the doctor's image, attitude and conduct. Did she meet your expectations, both professionally and personally?

Researchers form the School of Public and Environmental Affairs, Indiana University-Purdue University, Fort Wayne, Indiana conducted an interesting study that aimed to identify which attributes of a primary healthcare experience have the most impact on patient satisfaction. The study also tried to identify which aspects of each attribute were most significant in patients' response to the services they receive. Of the three attributes studied, *physician care* was most influential. It's all about perception, or at least that's what the psychiatrists claim. Somewhere deep in your mind you have an image of your doctor. You are more likely to trust the doctor if your previous expectations were met at least in part. In your perception, did the doctor care about you? Did you feel respect toward her?

Building trust with your physician requires both of you to participate, so if you opt out of participation, it's likely the trust may not last as long as it should. She may be a charming physician, but charm alone should not deceive your perception, as it is not enough for trust. Can she also deliver the care you expect to be trustworthy? A study by Thom and Kravitz at the University of California-San Francisco School of Medicine concluded that patients with a lower level of trust in their physician are more likely to report that requested or needed services are not provided.

The trust between you and your doctor is not meant to be blind; it needs eyes and ears for mutual participation. As long as you are mentally and psychologically capable of independence, the doctor should HELP you take care of yourself, rather than in the old days when the doctor would say, "I will take of you."

As my dad was a surgeon, I grew up watching lots of doctors. I have seen the molding process in medical school, listened to debates, and heard the ideas and dreams of many doctors, young and old. I came to believe that at the end of the process, many physicians love their profession, so they perform its duties and carry its burdens with passion while being excellent at what they do. But others are not that way. Just as the judge's gown can't guarantee a fair trial or a cop's uniform honesty, a white coat with an M.D. on it can't guarantee good medical care. Many doctors are good professionals but do health care as a job with no love and no passion, simply waiting for the weekend to come.

How you ultimately perceive the doctor should help you make the next move. Should you stick with that doctor, or find another one? Even if the interaction you just had with her was your first, it is probably good enough for you to figure out if you want her as your doctor. On the other hand if you've been going there for a while and can't make up your mind, think harder.

There's no question in my mind that if you want the most out of your doctor's visit(s) you have to like and trust her. The trust you have in your doctor will assure an important ingredient in health care called continuity of care. Continuity of your health care is important for you as a study by Donahue and Ashkin from the University of North Carolina concluded that *longer continuity of care was associated with greater patient satisfaction and confidence in one's physician.* If you are comfortable with your physician, that continuous relationship will pay big dividends as you get older.

The next step after you exit is to digest the information from your doctor.

Digest and Research

I know it's easy to blame medical jargon for your not understanding or misunderstanding the information given, but you still need to digest and research the information to achieve good results.

You want to digest the information you received during your visit, whether it was intended to protect your health (suggesting you stop smoking, eat a high fiber diet, exercise and so on) or to inform you of a problem (you have high blood pressure or you failed a hearing screen.) The information may be about your grade (success) in a care plan that was previously tailored for you—i.e. your blood sugar is still high, or the first course of antibiotics didn't eliminate your infection.

In the digestive system, big chunks of food are broken into smaller and smaller particles as they pass through. This process allows your body to absorb and benefit from every food item. If you remember the way I explained the final part of the SOAP, the plan "P" was loaded with items. You need to break up the chunks of information handed to you in the plan. The counseling part will tell you about the diagnosis, what is wrong with you, why it happened to you, and what you need to do to deal with it. The request for investigation will remind you of the missing pieces to confirm your diagnosis and solve the puzzle, grade the disease severity, or help with the management of your condition. The referral part will take you to higher levels of confidence about the diagnosis and the care plan, with hopefully both doctors agreeing on the same plan. And of course you need to digest and understand every instruction given about your medication.

In my practice, it's a little more challenging. I had a mother that brought four of her six children in yesterday, each for a different ailment. As each of them has a different age, weight, and diagnosis, I had to go over each one in detail. Two of the children had the exact same antibiotic and same dose, but different concentrations. Talk about this mother facing a challenge! Yet I've known her for years, and she's never failed.

When you care for more than one patient in your household, digest the information very slowly. Don't mix medication bottles or instructions as the consequences of misunderstanding or missing specific information can be serious.

I know for a fact that no one can accurately store all the information uploaded to his brain at the doctor's office via a broadband cable. Most likely you retain the title and headings, so now is the time to review the subject and material. I offer my patients handwritten or printed material for a reason, as I want to make sure that when they get home, they retain reminders of the plan. This is what I call Visual Aids.

My wife and kids laughed so hard watching one of the episodes of the hit TV show *Friends*. In that episode "Joey's" new roommate was mocking "Monica," saying "I see your lips move and all I can hear is *Blaa, Blaa, Blaa.*" Once in a while I look at my patient's eyes and facial expressions and wonder whether she's hearing and following me, or is it the Blaa, Blaa, Blaa. I try to get around the blaa, blaa, blaa effect by using visual aids, as two senses are better than one.

I found it very helpful in my daily practice to use visual aids to communicate with my patients and their parents. For example, instead of just talking about ear infections, I show them the diagram of the ear and its chambers and connections, then describe the difference between a middle ear versus an outer ear infection. Sometimes I show them the lung and airway on a three-dimensional model. I believe understanding what is wrong with you is a big part of the cure. When you feel you don't understand what your doctor is saying, ask her to draw or show you a diagram or a picture that will help you visualize the problem and understand it better. Also if you know the medical term for your problem, many of the health web sites will provide you with detailed and sometimes fascinating pictures. On a few occasions I've given the parents the name of the web site where I found informative photos and written down the medical diagnosis to shorten their search time.

I consider my use of visual aids as being in the primitive stage, as future doctors will have a lot more in their offices to offer their patients than we do now. They will have plasma TV screens, a medical database beyond the wildest imagination, 3D images, and software that will blow your mind away. As usual this technology will be descending to us from the top down. It is available now in large-budget, large-scale teaching hospitals, but as the prices drop and the technology improves, we in primary care will also be able to dazzle you with vivid pictures and illustrations. Who knows—you may actually enjoy your doctor's visit. Or better yet, be able to stay home as your Internet doctor will save you the trip by examining you in the comfort of your bedroom.

Why is researching and digesting the information important? Because research makes you a better consumer. You learn more about yourself and about health issues, if you recall the definition of serendipity as a fringe benefit of research. How long does it take you to research for a car or even car insurance? Did you ever buy a car from a dealer without researching the price, the specifications, the warranty (should I keep on going?)

You may not need to research all the items on your care plan menu, just the critical ones. Diagnosis, medications and treatment options are high on the list. Click on the mouse, enter the World Wide Web and type your diagnosis or the name of the medication. Select the web sites that sound professional. You don't have to waste time traveling all through the web, as 2 - 3 good web sites will be enough to validate and confirm your search.

First timers, as I call the first time parents, may need visual aid assurance even before they leave the office. As I was explaining the infant skin disease condition to his first time parents, I saw in their eyes the "I have no clue what you are talking about" look so I knew that if I didn't validate my speech, I would lose their cooperation in treating the disease. After I pulled a big oversized dermatology textbook, pointed at a picture that looked exactly like their child's rash, and read a few lines from the book with them, they were sold. They followed the plan of care to the end, and next time I saw the toddler he was cured.

There may not always be enough time for you to be sold on what your doctor told you in the office, but at the comfort and privacy of your home, there should be no excuse. This process of researching will help you get the most of your next doctor visit and allow you to be an active participant in taking care of your own health.

If you've been given a request for further investigation (blood work, X-ray), you may research the predictive value of those investigations when you are not convinced that it is needed. We use terms such as *positive predictive value* and *negative predictive value.* Those terms can translate into specificity and sensitivity of the investigation. If a test is highly sensitive and specific, it will confirm the diagnosis and put everyone's mind at ease. However, occasionally doctors order tests for different reasons.

When I first diagnose a child with asthma, I ask for a chest X-ray. However, during the long discussion, somewhere I mention that the X-ray won't prove or disprove my asthma diagnosis. Instead I'm asking for the chest X-ray to rule out other disorders. For some parents who try to take in all what I say at once, this explanation is missed. They call back and ask if the chest X-ray isn't for asthma, why do we have to do it? I repeat what I said before: that it is recommended to rule out the presence of other lung conditions that may imitate asthma. Is it important? Hundreds of chest doctors believe so. Go to their web site, http://www.chestnet.org/ and you will be able to find out why.

Each specialty and subspecialty in medicine has built a respectable informative web site. When you have a lung question, go to the chest physicians' web site and browse through the list of topics that interest you.

Researching medication is of particular importance as it has surfaced as an issue of major significance in health care. The list of medications is expanding faster than the ozone hole. The influx of data about old and new medication is overwhelming to all health professionals. Even if you do nothing else, you need to worry about the medication you've been given and look it up on the Internet. The local pharmacies now will give you a printout of basic information about your prescription, name, how to use it, and for how long. As the potential side effects are also included in the printout, try to read it when you get home.

Did you get the right medicine the doctor prescribed? Have you found out information about the drug that bothered you? Did you understand the why, the how and the what if about the drug? If you did, you are safer than those who did not.

Follow Up

By now, you either agreed with your PCP plan of care or not. If after thinking and researching, you're comfortable with his recommendation, you owe it to yourself to follow his advice. A mother of one of my patients told me yesterday, "I finally took him to a full evaluation and treatment of ADHD after you told me *you owe it to him as his mom to do what is best for his future.*"

Unfortunately I'm not that lucky all the time. Many times I've engaged with parents who agreed with everything I said, yet didn't follow my recommendation, not because they disagreed with me or mistrusted what I said. It was a *just because* kind of excuse.

One of my diabetic patients listened carefully to the whole lecture about his illness, risks, need for blood work to adjust his medication, all while his diabetic mother was showing me all the body language that I expected from full agreement. Yet it took me and my staff six weeks to get him to perform the needed blood work, he also missed two follow-up appointments and showed up to the third one sick enough to need more medication and lose more of his high school days. As a matter of fact when pediatricians and pediatric endocrinologists are asked about the most difficult group of diabetic patients to manage, the answer is likely adolescents. Although they show up to the appointment, listen, know how to test for blood sugar levels, and stay well informed about the medication dose, administration and adjustments, many end up in hospital emergency rooms with diabetic complications. Those are the ones who have a hard time following the care plan.

Let us say you're in perfect health and the follow-up plan is to come back in one year for another physical. Just remember the month in which you had your visit this year, as for annual physicals, exact dates aren't mandatory as long as you're checked once a year.

CONCLUSION

Let us stop here to recap.

Do you trust your doctor?
Yes   No
If yes, move to the next question; if no look for another doctor. You still have the original list of 3-5 primary care providers which now will again become useful.

Do you understand and agree with her plan?
Yes   Yes/but   No
If yes, move to the next question; if no or yes/but, call her back and ask for more information or clarification.

Are you willing to follow her recommendations?
Yes   No
If yes, you've won; if no, read this book through again.